Foreword

Much has happened since the first edition of *Consultant physicians working for patients* was published in 1999. Major media attention to a small number of high profile failures has damaged confidence in our system of health care. It is timely therefore to draw wider attention to the work that consultant physicians and this College are doing, in our determination to restore the trust between doctors and patients.

The report of the Bristol Royal Infirmary Inquiry puts the patient at the centre of health care, as we have long done implicitly if not explicitly. That report also states firmly that the safety of patients must be the foundation of quality. It emphasises that the components of care are much more than the actions or competence of health care professionals. They include working arrangements and relationships, with sound communication, and good physical environment and facilities. The recommendations of the report encompass clinical leadership and teamwork, standards of care and monitoring the quality of that care. Above all they reinforce the importance of close partnership with patients in making decisions about their care.

The inquiry report noted that in 2000 the present Government acknowledged finally the gap between rhetoric and reality in the NHS. A significant boost in funding was announced. A further commitment was made to align spending on the NHS with the average amount spent on health care in Europe. This development has been widely welcomed and is seen as a long-overdue recognition of the need for more resources.

These matters lie at the heart of this revised edition of *Consultant physicians working for patients*. The document sets out the views of the College on the conditions necessary for effective safe practice of internal medicine and its specialties in hospitals in the UK.

Part 1 reaffirms the duties and responsibilities of consultant physicians. It brings out more fully the changing conditions of the practice of medicine and the environment necessary for clinical excellence to flourish. It also reminds us of our duty to draw attention to shortcomings and failings that threaten the safety of patients. This part of the document gives particular attention to general internal medicine and the needs of patients who are acutely ill.

The document again emphasises the wide range of responsibilities that fall to consultants in their work to maintain and improve the quality of patient care. These responsibilities include teaching, training, research, continuing professional development and lifelong learning, clinical governance, and providing sound advice to managers and policy makers. Some of this work has an immediate impact upon patient care, but much represents the long-term investment in education and training, academic medicine and research upon which the future safety and quality of health care depend.

Part 2 contains statements on the specialties of medicine that the College represents. It describes the work of specialist physicians alongside their colleagues in many disciplines, and the facilities that are required to carry out this work. A chief aim of these statements is to inform and guide the preparation of job plans and the annual appraisal process, but they also serve a wider purpose. Each has been prepared by appropriate specialists and sometimes by the joint specialty committees. They may be referred to as position statements for the specialties. Although containing specialised information they should be readily understood by non-clinical colleagues and by those who represent patients. We also highlight the reasonable workload which should be expected of a consultant and emphasise the major strategies of consultants which pertain at present. We hope you find the revised, updated and improved version helpful.

November 2001

KGMM ALBERTI
President
Royal College of Physicians

Contents

Executive summary

This statement sets out the views of the Royal College of Physicians on the conditions necessary for effective practice of internal medicine and its specialties in hospitals in the UK. Its purpose is to inform discussion between physicians, clinical colleagues and health service managers on:

- the provision, organisation and delivery of services in internal medicine and its specialties;
- factors that determine the level of care that can be provided, its safety and quality;
- deficiencies that must be remedied to maintain the safety and quality of care; and
- the preparation of job plans for consultant physicians.

The document restates the nature of medical professionalism, and the qualities that patients expect in their doctors. It outlines the range of work that physicians do. Besides their chief task – the care of patients – physicians work to maintain and improve the safety, effectiveness and quality of care. This work encompasses teaching, training, research, continuing professional development and lifelong learning, clinical governance, and the provision of authoritative advice to managers and policy makers. All are necessary. The competing demands they make upon the time available to a consultant must be properly balanced.

Increasing numbers of acutely ill patients, alongside changes in the nature of clinical practice, have prompted new approaches to the organisation and delivery of care. Many patients are elderly. Often they have multiple problems in addition to the acute illness that led to referral. Some patients need extended specialised treatment, commonly within elaborate clinical management programmes. All acutely ill patients require specialist care, to ensure the best prospect of full recovery.

These varied needs have also generated new ways of working. Throughout the health service health professionals work in teams, with mutual respect for the knowledge, skills and judgement that each member of a team brings. Indeed, this expression of team working is a prerequisite of modern medical care. To ensure that they function well for patients, these more elaborate, more inclusive ways of working must operate with clear lines and boundaries of responsibility, and impeccable communication.

Such developments in no way change the conclusions of previous reports that there are far too few consultant physicians to provide the services patients expect and need, and there are major deficiencies in the facilities necessary for safe, effective clinical practice.

Finally, the statement draws together recommendations from recent reports and deliberations of working groups set up by the College, groups in which the views of wider constituencies were represented or sought.

Glossary

Acute care physician
A physician who concentrates on the first 24 hours of medical care of acutely ill patients.

Acute medicine
That part of general internal medicine (qv) concerned with the specialist management of adult patients of all ages with a wide range of medical conditions, who are admitted to hospital as emergencies.

General internal medicine (GIM)
The foundation of hospital medical practice. It encompasses acute medicine (qv) and the specialist inpatient and outpatient care of patients with multiple disorders or ill-defined conditions that do not clearly fall within the remit of any of the system- or organ-based specialties of medicine.

General physician
A physician who undertakes general internal medicine (qv). It is usual for a general physician also to be a specialist in one of the system- or organ-based specialties of medicine.

On-call (or **on call**)
This term signifies the duty of a senior doctor or member of the team to be available to respond to requests of colleagues to give advice on and, if necessary, to attend patients whose problems call for the specialised skills of that particular doctor and team. Those skills are usually those of the system- or organ-based specialties of medicine, in contrast to those of doctors *on take* (qv) who have responsibility for referrals of unselected acutely ill patients.

On-take (or **on take**)
The term *take* and its derivatives signify the duty of a senior doctor or member of the team to take responsibility for the care and management of acutely ill patients. Such patients are usually referred by a general practitioner, a colleague in the emergency department, the outpatient department or the inpatient wards of the hospital. The arrangement makes clear who is responsible for the prompt care of patients who are acutely ill, to minimise delay in providing appropriate and safe care.

Round
A round is the formal procedure when a senior doctor, usually a consultant but often a specialist registrar of considerable experience, and the clinical team, review patients who have entered an assessment ward or have been admitted to a main hospital ward.

Post-take rounds
These rounds are for the review of recent admissions of acutely ill patients. They are designed to ensure that acutely ill patients are assessed promptly by experienced physicians who can also secure ready access to other experienced opinion, with continuing review throughout the acute phase of illness.

Specialist
A physician with a specialty other than that of general internal medicine (qv).

Take (see **on-take**)

PART 1

DUTIES AND RESPONSIBILITIES

1 Introduction

1.1   This statement sets out the views of the Royal College of Physicians on the conditions necessary to serve patients well, through the effective practice of internal medicine and its specialties in hospitals in the UK. The chief purpose of the statement is to inform discussion between physicians, their clinical colleagues, health service managers and the health departments on:

- the provision, organisation and delivery of services in internal medicine and its specialties;
- factors that determine the level of patient care that can be provided;
- factors that determine the safety and quality of patient care;
- deficiencies that must be remedied to maintain the safety and quality of care; and
- the preparation of job plans for consultant physicians.

1.2   The statement also provides information for patient representatives and advocates.

1.3   Physicians do not work alone. The service they give to patients depends upon close collaboration with colleagues in many other specialties and disciplines. But this statement is drawn from the perspective of consultant physicians, to whom patients look for the maintenance of standards in their specialist and general medical care.

BACKGROUND

1.4   In 1999 the College published the first edition of *Consultant physicians working for patients*.[1] The document restated familiar, longstanding concerns that changes in the conditions of work of physicians continued to threaten the standards of clinical care they were able to give to patients.[2] It again drew attention to the increasing pressure of emergency admissions and the needs of acutely ill patients, alongside the rising demand for care by the specialised services of medicine. The effects on clinical care had been compounded by changes in the training and work patterns of junior medical staff, resulting in fewer experienced junior staff. The document pointed to the numerous other duties, in addition to direct patient care, that lay within the responsibilities of consultants.

1.5   It concluded, as had previous reports, that there were too few consultant physicians, working with insufficient staff, in facilities that too often were unsuitable for the task.

1.6   These concerns remain, although much work is being done to address them, both within and outside the College. Besides an unabated increase in the demand for care, there have been further changes in the conditions and provision of health care and its organisation; and there have been new developments in the regulation, oversight and responsibilities of the profession. In addition, the problems raised by an increasing amount of work with insufficient trained staff have stimulated examination of wider roles for health care staff.[3] The College has therefore undertaken a review and revision of the previous document.

1.7   This revised statement places the work of consultant physicians within the setting of their duties and responsibilities. It describes the work that consultants do, both in patient care and in activities to maintain and improve the quality of health care in this country. The topics are treated concisely but are supported by reference to essential documents, mostly from the College, the General Medical Council, and the government. The statement draws together the pertinent recommendations from the documents cited. A source of advice and information on related matters that lie outwith the chief remit of the College is *The Consultant Handbook,* produced by the Central Consultants and Specialists Committee.[4]

2 Medical professionalism

2.1   The first responsibility of the doctor is to the individual patient. This places the clinical consultation, with its elements of listening, examination, investigation, diagnosis and explanation, and therapeutic intervention at the heart of medical practice.[5] Furthermore, the clinical consultation respects the right of patients to participate fully in decisions on their care, ensuring they are sufficiently well informed to do so.[6,7]

2.2   Patients expect their doctors to be caring, compassionate individuals who have a broad knowledge of human behaviour, are empathic and are able to communicate in ways that assist understanding. The exercise of these attributes affirms the reality of partnership between doctor and patient.[8]

2.3   The advice doctors give is often qualified by uncertainty. Yet patients must have confidence in the knowledge, skill and conduct of doctors, and be able to place trust in their judgement and recommendations.

2.4   The special qualities that characterise the clinical consultation are sought by patients and their advocates, and are deeply ingrained in the professional ethos. Such are the professional obligations of doctor to patient that neglect of these qualities earns peer rebuke, public criticism, and sanction by the statutory bodies.[6]

2.5   By virtue of their learning and experience, and the investment in them that society has made, doctors also have a special part in the stewardship of our health care system. It is a role that carries wider duties and responsibilities, and further accountability. This has long been understood, but is now increasingly made explicit as the processes of health care and the work of health professionals within them become subject to closer scrutiny.

2.6   These wider duties and responsibilities are now identified much more clearly within the working arrangements of consultants. They should be specified in their contracts and job plans (see Part 2 of this document which contains descriptions of the work of consultants in the specialties and in Appendix 1 the templates for the preparation of job plans).

PROFESSIONAL REGULATION

2.7   The statutory right to self-regulation imposes great responsibilities on the profession, and every medical practitioner must be familiar with those responsibilities.[6] Doctors are required to observe the principles of *Good medical practice* and the standards of competence, care and conduct expected in all aspects of professional work. They should consider whether the care they provide accords with standards set by the General Medical Council, the medical Royal Colleges, and the specialist societies. Doctors must safeguard trust in those professional standards by being alert to risks to the welfare of patients. They must take proper action when they perceive such risks, or when things go wrong.

CONTINUING PROFESSIONAL DEVELOPMENT AND REVALIDATION

2.8   Doctors have a duty to keep their knowledge and skills up-to-date.[6] Consultants must now demonstrate, and not merely assert, the strength of their commitment to continuing professional development by accepting professional assessment, including regular peer review. Each year consultants are required to participate in an appraisal of their performance, a process that will also inform revalidation. With the greater emphasis now given, quite properly, to continuing professional development and professional appraisal, consultants must be able to put aside adequate protected time for this work. In fact, the Department of Health now requires that NHS employers recognise that preparation time and time for carrying out the appraisal replace, rather than supplement, the consultant's existing duties and workload, and that employers explicitly release consultants from other duties for a specified period. A responsibility also falls on employing trusts to support study leave and to provide access to continuing professional development.

2.9   The programme of continuing professional development should reflect the whole range of work of a physician. It should therefore include time specifically focused on general medicine besides the specialty interest, and also the wide range of other professional activities that a physician is required to undertake.

3 Work of consultant physicians

EMPLOYMENT OF CONSULTANTS

3.1   Almost all consultants are employed by NHS trusts under terms and conditions of service that are negotiated nationally and locally through formal mechanisms.[4] A significant number of consultants have a substantive appointment with an NHS trust or a university and have an honorary contract with the other. These matters lie outwith the remit of the College, except insofar as standards of clinical practice and quality of care may be influenced by them.

JOB PLANS

3.2   The job plan is a statement of the duties and responsibilities of a consultant, the activities they generate and the resources and facilities needed to carry them out. The job plan should include a work programme, which quantifies the work. There is detailed guidance on the preparation of job plans in Part 2 of this document.

WAYS OF WORKING

Medical teams   3.3   Although consultants are accountable for their conduct and practice individually, they do not work in isolation. Throughout the health service they work in teams, with mutual respect for the knowledge, skills and judgement that each member of a team brings.[6] Indeed, this expression of team working is a prerequisite of modern medical care.[9]

3.4   Except in one crucial respect – the role of consultants in leadership – the team has long ceased to resemble the small close-knit medical firm of the past.[2] It is an extended body and is multiprofessional and multidisciplinary. The changed conditions of work of individual members mean that its composition – including the complement of junior doctors – is ever changing. Nonetheless, the term is usefully kept to describe the small group of people who work together regularly. Such a team depends for its effectiveness upon strong clinical leadership, firm clinical alliances with members of other teams, and good communication within and between teams.

Multiprofessional and multidisciplinary working   3.5   Participation of a wide range of health professionals in the care of individual patients is normal practice in many services; for example, in services for the health care of elderly people,[10] in services for diabetes, and in nutrition support teams. More recently it has been examined in relation to cancer services[11] and in management of stroke, where there is evidence that organised multidisciplinary care does improve outcome.[12]

3.6   Multidisciplinary team working may be made more effective by adoption of agreed policies and practices, standardised treatments and joint training programmes. New service models seek to exploit the potential benefits that collective professional assessment, review, and decision-making can bring. If decision-making is subject to continuing peer review, clinical management should be less variable, and the findings of research more promptly assimilated into practice.

3.7   There have been similar, specific applications of these approaches to other services; for example, in joint case management between gastroenterologists and surgeons in gastrointestinal bleeding. Even more familiar are the systems of integrated care – across primary and secondary care – that have been adopted in the management of common chronic disorders; for example, diabetes and asthma.

3.8   The form of service delivery described as a managed clinical network aims to bring a unified specialist service to populations larger than those normally served by a single institution or administrative area.[11] It too espouses multidisciplinary working, seeking to give unbroken care to individuals served by the network, regardless of where each element of care is delivered.

Changing responsibilities

3.9   Broader corporate approaches to clinical decision-making offer benefits for patients; but dispersal of responsibility from a particular consultant – the patient's physician – does have implications for clinical practice and the responsibilities of consultants.[13]

3.10   These approaches highlight the importance of the processes of delivery of care. They remind us that sources of medical error most often lie in the failure of systems, and of processes involving several people rather than the failure of an individual clinician.[14] Inadequate documentation and poor communication are particular causes of error or adverse events.[15] To ensure that these more elaborate, more inclusive ways of working function well for patients, they must operate with clear lines and boundaries of responsibility.

3.11   The movement of traditional professional boundaries invites a fresh look at the work of consultant physicians and other doctors, to consider whether some activities should be transferred to other health staff, to make more medical time available for patients.[3]

Sequential care – the journey of care

3.12   Even in hospital, patients often do not remain in the care of one team. Patients admitted as emergencies need effective specialist management of acute illness in the first instance. They might not remain the responsibility of the team that first receives them, but pass into the care of other teams having the different skills and expertise needed for further care, and then to other, more appropriate forms of care – the journey of care (see Chapter 4).

Consultants working with general practitioners

3.13   Besides their formal roles within hospital, many consultants make themselves accessible for direct consultation with general practitioners. This relationship enriches the quality of care, which may be further enhanced when consultants hold clinics in primary care.

Consultants working with patients

3.14   The medical problems and needs of individual patients lie at the heart of the work of doctors. Physicians are well placed, therefore, to strengthen the partnership between patients and professional staff. Consultants are members of the boards and advisory structures of charitable organisations, and they contribute to the work of patient support groups (although this kind of work normally lies outwith service contracts).

3.15   In the Royal College of Physicians there is a Patients and Carers Liaison Committee. The committee was set up to ensure that the interests of patients and informal carers are fully represented in the work of the College. There are similar arrangements in most NHS trusts.

Consultants supporting consultants

3.16   Established consultants have long seen it as a professional duty to mentor their newly appointed colleagues, and to be available as informal sources of advice, tutorship and support. The New Consultants Committee of the College may have a role in promoting the development of local professional support networks to enable this duty to be performed effectively.

Summary points

WAYS OF WORKING [3.3–3.16]

Medical teams – Consultants work in teams, which are multiprofessional and multidisciplinary. The effectiveness of teams depends on strong clinical leadership, firm clinical alliances with members of other teams, and good communication within and between teams.

Multiprofessional and multidisciplinary working [3.5–3.11] – Participation of a wide range of health professionals in the care of individual patients is increasingly common. Such working may be strengthened by adoption of agreed policies and practices, standardised treatments and joint training programmes.

Managed clinical networks aim to bring a unified specialist service to populations larger than those normally served by a single institution or administrative area. They too espouse multidisciplinary working, seeking to give unbroken care to individuals served by the network, wherever each element of care is delivered.

Corporate approaches to clinical decision offer benefits for patients, but dispersal of responsibility does have implications for clinical practice and the responsibilities of consultants. To ensure that they function well for patients, these more elaborate, more inclusive ways of working must operate with clear lines – and boundaries – of responsibility.

Sequential care – the journey of care [3.12] – Patients often do not remain in the care of one team. Patients admitted as emergencies need effective specialist management of acute illness first. They may pass into the care of other teams having the different skills and expertise needed for further care; and then pass to other, more appropriate forms of care – the journey of care.

Consultants working with general practitioners [3.13] – Besides their formal roles within hospital, many consultants make themselves accessible for direct consultation with general practitioners. This relationship enriches the quality of care.

Consultants working with patients [3.14–3.15] – The medical problems and needs of individual patients lie at the heart of the work of doctors. Physicians are well-placed to strengthen the partnership between patients and professional staff.

Consultants working for consultants [3.16] – Established consultants have long seen it as a professional duty to mentor their newly appointed colleagues and to be available as informal sources of advice, tutorship and support.

4 General internal medicine and its specialties

4.1   Before the trend to specialisation, although many consultant physicians developed an expertise in their chosen areas, most practised general internal medicine and dealt with a wide range of medical problems. These included patients admitted as emergencies, patients with multiple disorders, patients referred to outpatient clinics for investigation and diagnosis, and patients referred by specialist services – as outpatients or urgent inpatient referrals.

MEDICAL SPECIALISATION

4.2   Better understanding of the mechanisms of disease, and advances in clinical management – such as the introduction of refined investigative and therapeutic techniques that require new skills and experience – have promoted increasing specialisation in medicine. This has led to further progress, with improved outcomes for patients.[16] Patients expect specialists to be closely involved in their care. Higher medical training, in its content and duration, has increasingly been fashioned to meet the requirement for specialists. Unsurprisingly, specialisation has influenced the training and practice of other groups of health professionals.

4.3   The specialties of medicine, of which there are now over twenty, are described in Part 2.

ACUTE AND EMERGENCY MEDICINE

4.4   With progressive differentiation of the medical specialties fewer physicians feel able to undertake general, acute and emergency work in addition to other specialised work for which training has prepared them. Yet alongside the development of new specialties, hospital practice has seen increasing numbers of patients referred for acute medical care, mostly as emergencies. The benefits that have come from advances in specialist care[16] must be matched by excellence in emergency care.[17]

4.5   Referral for acute medical care is an increasingly large part of consultant medical work. Patients admitted urgently or as emergencies now occupy 70–80% of medical beds – nearer 95% in some district hospitals.[18] Most of these patients are elderly. Besides the illness for which they require acute care, many have chronic disorders and multiple pathologies that cause disability.

4.6   Whatever their age, patients need and expect effective specialist management of acute illness. They may also have problems that require the expertise of other specialists. Often they need the skills of assessment, rehabilitation and re-enablement that are expected of a comprehensive geriatric service. Thus, the care of many patients referred with acute medical problems requires a coherent multispecialty, multidisciplinary approach.[10] This has implications for the organisation of acute care. These implications are considered below.

4.7   Currently about half of the 6,343 consultant physicians in the UK participate in the take* of acute unselected admissions. Specialists in cardiology, diabetes and endocrinology, gastroenterology, geriatrics and respiratory medicine, for example, spend 40–60% of their time in the management of patients who are admitted as emergencies, on take. Consultants in other medical specialties also spend a significant proportion of their time in this work. Physicians and their teams who undertake this work must be skilled and experienced in the diagnosis and management of the common conditions besides those of their specialty.

4.8   Many elderly patients come under the care of specialist teams other than geriatrics. Drawing upon the multidisciplinary skills of the geriatric service can improve the success of care. Similarly, elderly patients under the care of geriatricians might also require other specialist advice on the conditions that contributed to their admission. The report *Management of the older medical patient*[10] gives a comprehensive account of the care of the older medical patient.

4.9   The requirements for safe effective care of patients who are admitted as emergencies have raised important questions about the provision and organisation of emergency care and about the training and continuing professional development of physicians who undertake this care. The issues are treated comprehensively in *Acute medicine: the physician's role.*[18]

4.10   It is the view of the College that skill in general medicine, including acute medicine, is integral to all specialties that manage acute problems. To ensure that physicians are competent in acute care there should be unified training in general internal medicine, including acute elements, across the medical specialties.[18] In keeping with this approach the appointment of physicians solely to provide acute care without links to a specialty or an adequate infrastructure for acute care should be discouraged. (However, there are now over 20 full-time acute care physicians in the UK, with non-standard job descriptions and variable posts and very differently organised jobs. Individual post-holders seem to have met a real need to improve the quality of acute care in their own hospitals.)

ORGANISATION OF ACUTE CARE

4.11   The safety and effectiveness of care are much influenced by the organisation and working of the service.[19] This is true of the care given to all patients but is crucially so for those who are admitted urgently or as emergencies. Any hospital that receives such patients must provide emergency care with comprehensive investigative, patient monitoring and treatment services – including surgical services – for 24 hours every day.

4.12   Each stage of care requires professional staff with special skills, acting in concert. The safe passage of a patient from one stage to another depends on formal arrangements for transfer of responsibility. These arrangements must be punctiliously observed, with faultless communication within and between teams. The point is so important as to warrant repetition in this document.

---

*See glossary

Accident and emergency (A&E) departments

4.13   There are about 13 million A&E attendances each year. About 3 million follow a 999 call, and 1 million are referred by their general practitioner. About 9 million attend without prior professional assessment. Of all these patients, 80–85% return home that day, 70–80% having suffered minor trauma.

4.14   Many of the 3.9 million patients each year who are admitted as medical emergencies are received via the A&E department. Usually this follows an initial assessment by their general practitioner and the referral is made to the on-take* medical team. Some ill patients are admitted from the outpatient clinic and others are admitted following arrival and assessment in A&E. Where a specialist team already knows the patient, direct admission under that team is often judged best. Other acutely ill medical patients are brought to A&E by ambulance in response to a 999 call. These medical patients are a minority (15–20%) of all those who arrive at A&E departments, but they include many of the most seriously ill.

4.15   A small number of this diverse group of people have illness or trauma requiring immediate, life-saving measures. More have other serious conditions that command prompt attention by clinicians who are skilled and experienced in the assessment and management of various kinds of trauma and illness. In about 5% there are compounding social or mental problems. But most patients are found to have relatively minor problems and do not require the whole range of skills and facilities of a comprehensive emergency department. The need for prompt, safe assessment of every patient, to ensure that each receives appropriate care, presents a major challenge to emergency services and their organisation.

4.16   The services required by patients who come to the A&E department encompass prompt initial assessment, resuscitation, major trauma care, acute medical care, intensive care, and coronary care, supported by comprehensive investigative services. It is self-evident that these services should be closely linked and co-located. The issues surrounding emergency care are the subject of much deliberation and debate.[18,20] They extend beyond the scope of this statement, indeed beyond the activities of the A&E department, but they bear closely upon the work of physicians and medical teams. However, it is widely accepted that the diverse needs of such a variety of patients call for an integrated approach to their reception, initial and subsequent assessment and clinical management. This implies a careful new appraisal of the range of health professional skills that should be available in the A&E department, and the staff who should have them.

Medical assessment units and medical admission units

4.17   These matters have generated innovative practical responses.[18,20,21] Medical assessment units (observation areas) and medical admission units have been set up. They serve to minimise delay between initial assessment of patients and bringing them into the care of a medical team that is prepared for them. (Note that these terms, and the term *alpha ward,* have been applied in different ways to describe arrangements for the assessment, observation and initial care of patients with acute problems.[20]) Dedicated facilities of this kind should be operated in close collaboration with the emergency department.

4.18   A *medical assessment unit* provides close monitoring of patients before a decision is made either to admit them to a medical ward or refer them to other forms of care. Medical assessment units facilitate early comprehensive appraisal of the complex problems of older people (providing a forum for contact with social services and community teams). It

*See glossary

provides a way of making sure that old people receive the care that is appropriate for them, do not go to intermediate care unless that is appropriate, and perhaps even spares them unnecessary admission.[22]

4.19   A *medical admission unit* is a ward to which patients are admitted for immediate treatment and continuing assessment, and from which – within 24 hours preferably, or a few days at most – they are transferred to a medical ward for appropriate specialist or other forms of care. Gathering acutely ill patients into a single area is safer. It enables continuing close observation by clinical staff familiar with these problems. Ready access to near patient investigation and consultant presence should aid diagnosis and institution of correct clinical management, including referral for further opinion. Such arrangements ease the conduct of in-take* and post-take* consultant rounds.*

4.20   The units are also places for a vital element of professional teaching and training, and must incorporate an area designed for this work.

4.21   Medical assessment and medical admission units require sufficient nurses to manage a high throughput of acutely ill patients. Some nurses and other non-medical staff will have extended roles and be skilled in investigative and therapeutic procedures including venesection, arterial blood sampling, electrocardiography, and bladder catheterisation.

Management of medical assessment units and medical admission units

4.22   The management structure must take account of the need for an acute general physician to be appointed to give clinical leadership and to take responsibility for the organisation, work practices and further development of a medical assessment or medical admission unit. It has been suggested that, provided they have links to a specialty and an adequate infrastructure for acute care, consultants in acute medicine might have such a role. Sessional time should be allocated for this work.

Intensive care medicine and A&E medicine

4.23   In 1999 the Department of Health set up a review of adult critical care services. The report, *Comprehensive critical care,*[23] describes a new approach to the delivery of services based upon severity of illness. In this sense, the existing division into high dependency and intensive care beds is to be replaced by a classification that focuses on the level of care that individual patients need. The document also recognised that the emergence of intensive care as a multidisciplinary specialty would involve the development of training schemes through which individuals aiming to practice within the acute medical specialties might pass at SHO or SpR level. For those choosing a career in intensive care medicine, a CCST will be available.

4.24   These developments have important implications for the organisation of the delivery of services to the acutely ill patient, and especially to the way physicians working in acute general medicine interact with the multidisciplinary teams, which are based principally within the intensive care unit and the accident and emergency department. The ways in which such services may be developed are currently under discussion by an RCP Working Party.

*See glossary

INTEGRITY OF CARE

Risk factors for adverse events

4.25   Many emergency patients are referred to hospital without a firm diagnosis. Scrutiny of adverse events in relation to medical emergencies has shown that errors in diagnosis and interpretation of investigative findings, and inadequate treatment and care, are frequently associated with factors that may be avoidable.[24,25] Among them are delayed consultant involvement, and failure to obtain other specialist opinion – especially experienced surgical opinion, but also that of colleagues in investigative specialties besides those in other medical specialties. Another notable factor is failure to use accepted treatment protocols for common conditions. Others are inadequate record keeping and poor communication.[15]

Consultant presence

4.26   The evidence reinforces the need for prompt assessment of these patients by experienced physicians who, by their authority, can secure ready access to other experienced opinion. There is a need for continuing review of ill patients throughout the acute phase, and finally, before discharge.[19]

4.27   There must always be consultant cover for an acute service. When a colleague provides leave cover, non-acute clinical sessions must be displaced. Naturally such arrangements should be planned in advance.

The medical team

4.28   A medical team should contain enough doctors of sufficient experience to manage the clinical work for which the consultant has responsibility. It should comprise a consultant and at least three resident staff (a specialist registrar, senior house officer (SHO), and house officer (HO), or two SHOs and a HO). Where consultants are on-call without a registrar, a member of the resident team who has completed general professional training and who preferably holds full MRCP(UK) should be available.

4.29   The evidence supports the case for ensuring that physicians who are freed from other responsibilities are readily available to lead, guide and support the on-take team, and to teach on the management of medical emergencies. In practice, because there are too few consultants, most keep their fixed outpatient sessions, and at the same time provide cover both for their junior colleagues who receive and assess emergency referrals and those with responsibility for ward patients. This is not satisfactory.

4.30   The unpredictability and intensity of emergency referral calls for the undivided attention of the medical team. There must be separate junior medical cover for patients in the wards who have ongoing medical problems and for surgical patients requiring medical care. Similarly, specialty work in outpatients must not clash with the care of patients who are acutely ill.

4.31   Last, junior doctors must be confident that they can call on senior colleagues at any time, and will receive unreserved support.

Consultant led in-take and post-take rounds

4.32   The purposes of these rounds are to improve the safety and quality of care, and to reinforce leadership, support and guidance to junior doctors. They are also teaching rounds. Because of the intensity of take and post-take work it may be necessary for consultants to hold separate post-take teaching rounds for students.

4.33   The consultant on take must become familiar with the medical and social background of each patient, verify the clinical findings, review the results of investigations and agree further management. Patients rightly expect the consultant with responsibility for their care to explain events to them and to their relatives, and to give sufficient time to this.

4.34   The College recommends that a consultant should carry out a post-take round with the team. Patients admitted as emergencies should be reviewed at least every 24 hours by a consultant or by a specialist registrar (with a consultant available at all times) and more often if there are concerns about patients or the intake is large.

Acute illness load

4.35   The attention that the medical team must give to each acutely ill patient places a limit on the number who can be cared for safely. The College remains of the view that over a 24-hour period the consultant and team should not be expected to take responsibility for more than 20–25 acutely ill patients. When these levels are exceeded frequently, the team should be limited to 12 hours on-take or there should be two teams. Neither should they be required to participate in the acute rota more often than one day in five. Similarly, a medical team should not be responsible for more than 25 inpatients. Larger numbers and unrelieved pressure threaten patient safety, besides the quality of care. For the same reasons a consultant should not normally work single-handed in the major medical specialties that are involved in acute medicine.

Serving relatives and carers

4.36   This statement has emphasised the central place of the clinical consultation, whether in measured or urgent circumstances. Relatives and carers, too, seek access to the doctor. They make a further call upon that scarce resource – consultant time. But without sufficient time, given without reserve or distraction, the quality of the encounter is at risk. Those who are not ill, but are worried nonetheless, also need the doctor's time, for thoughtful explanation and reassurance; and they need to feel at ease, knowing that this is a proper call upon the service and the doctors within it. At present this cannot be achieved regularly, because of the shortage of consultant staff.

CONTINUITY OF CARE

4.37   Continuity of care is crucial to its safety and quality. Unless essential conditions are met the journey of the acutely ill patient from arrival, through initial assessment, admission and subsequent passage through specialist or multispecialty care, may be perilous.

4.38   The College reiterates the need for impeccable communication within and between teams when responsibility for patients is transferred. It is best if there is a formal transfer, for which time is set aside.

4.39   Unfortunately, the requirement to reduce the hours of work of junior doctors has resulted in some of them necessarily working shifts and partial shifts. In these circumstances there is a threat to continuity in the care of acutely ill patients, both during intake and subsequently. This threatens not only the quality of care but also that of teaching and training.

4.40   Patients rightly expect the same quality of clinical care at weekends – including the long holiday weekends – as at any other time. This will usually require transfer of responsibility between consultants and between members of teams. The transfer should include a review of ill patients. In addition, the changing team must be ready to deal with unexpected relapses and must have ready access to consultant opinion at all times. In order to maintain safety of care, besides consultants there must be enough junior doctors to avoid infringement of the Working Time Directive. Each medical department should draw up and agree a formal plan to ensure the review of ill patients over a long weekend.

RESOURCES AND PROVISION FOR ACUTE CARE

4.41   The increasing number of emergency referrals to hospital has highlighted major shortcomings in the provision of care. A common, familiar problem is that there are too few serviced beds, and often those that are available are badly located and inappropriately serviced for the clinical need. However, the critical factor is that there are too few physicians and too few nurses. This is most evident when acutely ill patients are admitted.

Efficiency of care   4.42   Emergency outpatient clinics can ease the demand for emergency admission, especially if supported by access to fast track investigative services. But there are too few of them.[18]

4.43   Undoubtedly some patients are admitted for acute hospital care who might have been spared admission but for the lack of more appropriate facilities in the community. Similarly a better managed flow of patients to more appropriate forms of care, following satisfactory recovery from the acute episode, would ease the familiar delays experienced by newly admitted patients.[18]

OUTPATIENT CLINICS

4.44   Much of the non-acute work of the specialties of medicine is conducted in the outpatient department. Although few of the conditions encountered in that setting require immediate treatment, there is often a need to reach a prompt diagnosis. The College therefore believes that there should be close supervision of trainee doctors in the outpatient department, and that it should be normal practice to review selected cases at the end of a clinic, both for the safety of patients and for teaching and learning.

4.45   The College recognises that there may be occasions when the consultant will not be present in the outpatient clinic, and accepts that if such sessions were to be cancelled the service would be compromised. In these circumstances, the necessary supervision may be achieved in several ways:

▌ There may be cross-over from a consultant colleague who is in the hospital, and is available for advice. Ideally this cover would be in the same specialty, though this might not be possible in small hospitals. Advice may be given by telephone.

▌ Specialist registrars require different levels of advice, according to their experience and seniority. Debriefing following a trainee-run clinic is the minimum acceptable level of supervision. It may also be necessary to discuss the clinic list beforehand.

▌ An experienced clinical assistant, staff grade doctor or associate specialist may also provide support and back-up, but not as an alternative to consultant supervision.

4.46   An outpatient clinic should be cancelled if otherwise pre-MRCP doctors would be left without direct supervision.

INFORMATION TO SUPPORT PATIENT CARE

Patient information at admission   4.47   For optimal management it is essential that the most recent and relevant patient records and information are available promptly. This is a risk management issue and requires adequate administrative systems and efficient management of the admissions process.

The continuing clinical record

4.48   Doctors have a responsibility to keep clear, accurate and complete records of patient care.[6] Safe, effective care depends upon these records. The evidence is that too often they are poor; therefore consultants have a duty to lead by example.

4.49   Clinical records also have an essential place in learning and understanding, and they provide a focus for professional education and clinical audit. Inevitably clinical records become a matter of close interest in the response to patients' and relatives' complaints.

Patient information at discharge

4.50   The need for continuity of care at the time of discharge from hospital also requires good communication. The referring general practitioner must be advised promptly and sufficiently of the outcome of referral. Accurate documentation of the procedures carried out and the diagnosis is essential for good patient care,[26] and should be agreed by the whole team, prior to discharge. Again this is a risk management issue, and reinforces the important role of an experienced, full-time personal secretary or personal assistant within the team (see 5.2 also).

4.51   The wider issues of data collection and management, and information technology in the NHS, are considered briefly in Chapter 5.

Summary points and recommendations

MEDICAL SPECIALISATION [4.1–4.3]

Medical progress has promoted specialisation in medicine, with improved outcomes for patients. Patients expect specialists to be closely involved in their care. Higher medical training, in its content and duration, has increasingly been fashioned to meet the requirement for specialists.

ACUTE AND EMERGENCY MEDICINE [4.4–4.10]

Patients admitted urgently or as emergencies occupy 70-80% of medical beds. Most are elderly. All need specialist management of their acute illness, besides problems that require the expertise of other specialists.

The College *recommends* that:

▌ to protect the quality of acute medical care, more physicians are trained in general internal medicine, including acute medicine, in addition to a specialty.

▌ since many acutely ill medical patients are elderly, the multispecialty and multidisciplinary skills of assessment and rehabilitation that are characteristic of a comprehensive geriatric service should be available to complement acute care.

ORGANISATION OF ACUTE CARE [4.11–4.24]

Hospitals that receive acutely ill patients must provide emergency care with comprehensive investigative, monitoring and treatment services, for 24 hours, every day; and they must ensure that there are sufficient medical and nursing staff consultants trained and experienced in the care of these patients.

Summary points and recommendations – continued

Accident and emergency departments [4.13–4.16] – The services required by patients who come to the A&E department range from primary care to life-saving interventions. It is widely accepted that such diverse needs call for an integrated approach to the reception of patients, their assessment and clinical management. There is much discussion about the organisation of this service, its staffing and their training needs.

Medical assessment units and medical admission units [4.17–4.22] – These units provide for the safe care of acutely ill patients, with quality and efficiency, and are a resource for teaching in the management of acute illness.

The College *recommends* that:

▌ there should be a dedicated facility, operated in close collaboration with the accident and emergency department, for the assessment and/or admission of acute medical emergencies. It should have the necessary infrastructure and nursing staff – some with extended roles – to manage a high throughput of acutely ill patients.

▌ an acute general physician should be appointed to give leadership, and to take responsibility for the organisation, work practices and further development of the unit.

▌ arrangements are made for impeccable liaison within the unit and between the unit and other teams and departments, to ensure coordination of many elements of care, and the safe passage of a patient through further stages of care.

▌ the unit is the place for a vital element of professional teaching and training, and must incorporate an area designed for this work.

Intensive care medicine and A&E medicine [4.23–4.24] – New developments have implications for the organisation of the delivery of services to the acutely ill patient and for the way physicians working in acute general medicine interact with the teams based principally within the intensive care unit and the A&E department.

INTEGRITY OF CARE [4.25–4.36]

Consultant presence – The evidence supports the case for ensuring that consultant physicians who are experienced in acute medicine are readily available to participate in the work of the acute medical team.

The College *recommends* that arrangements are made:

▌ to ensure that consultant physicians – freed from other responsibilities – are readily available to lead, guide and support the on-take team, and to teach on the management of medical emergencies.

▌ to provide for cancellation of conflicting duties – including those that are normally fixed – when physicians cross cover for colleagues in acute medicine.

The medical team – Emergency referral calls for undivided attention.

The College *recommends* that arrangements are made:

▌ for separate junior medical cover for patients in the wards who have medical problems.

▌ to ensure that specialty work in outpatients does not clash with the care of patients who are acutely ill.

Summary points and recommendations – continued

Emergency take and post-take rounds – Acutely ill patients should be assessed promptly by experienced physicians who can secure ready access to other experienced opinion, with continuing review throughout the acute phase.

The College *recommends* that:

- a consultant should carry out a post-take round with the team.
- patients admitted as emergencies should be reviewed at least every 24 hours by a consultant or specialist registrar (with consultant available at all times) and more often if there are concerns about patients or the intake is large.
- arrangements should be made to cancel a consultant physician's other formal duties when an acute take round is due; and to cancel or modify clinics and technical lists that fall immediately after a period of acute on-call medicine.

Clinical load – The safety, quality and efficiency of patient care, and the quality of teaching, are affected by the workload.

The College *recommends* that:

- the consultant and team should not be expected to take responsibility for more than 20–25 acutely ill patients over a 24-hour period. When these levels are exceeded frequently, the team should be limited to 12 hours on take or there should be two teams.
- a medical team should not be responsible for more than 25 inpatients.
- the acute on-call rota should be no more than one day in five.
- a consultant should not normally work single-handed in a hospital in the major medical specialties.

CONTINUITY OF CARE [4.37–4.40]

Continuity of care is crucial to its safety and quality.

The College *recommends* that:

- there should be an arrangement in place to ensure flawless communication within and between teams when responsibility for patients is transferred. This is vital when the transfer is between members of the same team as they change periods of duty, or from one team to another.
- each medical department should draw up and agree a formal plan to ensure the review of ill patients over a long weekend.

RESOURCES AND PROVISION FOR ACUTE CARE [4.41–4.43]

There are major shortcomings in provision. Often there are too few appropriately serviced beds in the right place. But the critical factor is that there are too few physicians and too few nurses (see Chapter 7).

Efficiency of care – Meanwhile the College *recommends* that trusts and health authorities explore measures that could improve the efficiency of care without jeopardising quality. For example:

- with appropriate facilities in the community some patients might be spared hospital admission.
- primary care would be helped by readier access to investigations and emergency outpatient clinics.
- a better managed flow of patients to more appropriate forms of care, anticipating recovery from the

Summary points and recommendations – continued

acute episode, and subsequent health and social care needs, would ease delays experienced by newly admitted patients.

OUTPATIENT CLINICS [4.44–4.46]

The College *recommends* that:

▍ there should be close supervision of trainee doctors in the outpatient department, both for the safety of patients and for teaching and learning.

▍ an outpatient clinic should be cancelled if otherwise pre-MRCP doctors would be left without direct supervision.

INFORMATION TO SUPPORT PATIENT CARE [4.48–4.51]

Patient information at admission – For optimal management it is essential that the most recent and relevant patient information is available promptly. This is a risk management issue and requires adequate administrative systems and efficient management of the admissions process.

The College *recommends* that:

▍ the current medical records of patients <u>must</u> be available at the time they are admitted.

The continuing clinical record – Safe effective care depends upon clear, accurate and complete clinical records. The evidence is that too often they are poor.

The College *recommends* that:

▍ consultants have a duty to lead by example in keeping good clinical records.

Patient information at discharge – Continuity of care at discharge from hospital requires good communication between team, patient and referring doctor. The referring general practitioner should be advised promptly and sufficiently of the outcome of referral. An experienced personal assistant is essential for making these links.

The College *recommends* that:

▍ the clinical team must include an experienced personal secretary or personal assistant at the proper level (see also 5.2).

5 Supporting staff and facilities

CONSULTANT'S OFFICE

5.1   There are general facilities and support that all consultants need to carry out their clinical duties. Each must have an office which allows the privacy necessary for conversations with professional colleagues, patients and relatives, and in which confidential papers are secure.

MEDICAL SECRETARY/PERSONAL ASSISTANT

5.2   There should be an experienced, full-time personal secretary or personal assistant at a level that fully recognises their skills and responsibilities. This person is an essential member of the clinical team, necessary for its professional working (see also 4.47).

CLINICAL INFORMATION SYSTEMS

5.3   The first purpose of clinical information systems is to support patient care. Secondary purposes include activity analysis, performance review, service planning, health surveillance, monitoring, clinical enquiry, and clinical audit. All are germane to clinical governance. Much of the available data on hospital activity, from which, for example, clinical indicators of quality and performance are derived, are poor. Case-mix data especially are inadequate. These data (Hospital Episode Statistics – HES) are derived from clinical information contained in the medical records of patients.[27] The validity of data derived from them depends upon the quality of this clinical information, and its coding, and the preparation of returns. Consultants have a responsibility to ensure that their junior staff maintain the medical notes in a way that eases the task of coding staff (see also 4.45).

5.4   The safe care of patients requires ready access to up-to-date information and reliable means of communication. Clinicians cannot rely upon paper records being available when they are needed. The effective introduction and use of agreed policies and practices, and of standardised management protocols, cannot be assured without information technology. Provision of this technology in many hospital trusts is inadequate. A particular weakness is the inability to communicate well between hospital departments.

5.5   An ambitious National Information Strategy, *Information for health*,[28] will support the National Performance Framework for the NHS.[29] The intention is that there should be a modern health information system with electronic records for every patient, capable of covering clinical indicators and even outcomes. It is unlikely that this goal will be reached for many years.

Recommendations

SUPPORTING STAFF AND FACILITIES [5.1–5.5]

Consultant's office [5.1–5.2]

The College *recommends* that:

▌ each consultant should have an office which allows the privacy necessary for conversations with professional colleagues, patients and relatives, and in which confidential papers are secure.

▌ the consultant should have an experienced, full-time personal secretary or personal assistant at a level that fully recognises their skills and responsibilities.

▌ This individual is an essential member of the clinical team, necessary for its professional working (see also 4.47).

Clinical information systems [5.3–5.5] – The safe and efficient care of patients requires ready access to up-to-date information and reliable means of communication. The effective introduction and use of agreed policies and practices, as well as standardised management protocols cannot be assured without information technology. Provision of information technology in many hospital trusts is inadequate.

The College *recommends* that:

▌ hospital information systems be much improved to support the safe care of patients.

6 Work to maintain and improve the quality of health care

PROFESSIONAL RESPONSIBILITIES IN EDUCATION, TRAINING AND ASSESSMENT

6.1   Doctors are not only charged with personal lifelong professional development, they also have duties and responsibilities in the education and training of those who follow them.[6, 30, 31] Consultants support, supervise, and contribute to the education, training and assessment of medical students and junior doctors. This is done both in the context of normal clinical work and in formal teaching, usually as part of structured programmes.

6.2   Newer ways of learning have not displaced traditional learning in the context of patient care. Unfortunately, other pressures upon consultants, and changes in the working conditions of doctors in training, have reduced the time and opportunity for this aspect of learning. There is no substitute for hands-on experience under skilled supervision, especially during the reception and management of patients with acute, often undiagnosed illness. The skills and learning acquired by students and doctors in training depend greatly upon the quality of their teachers, and their example.

6.3   Most undergraduate teaching is done by NHS consultants, and a significant amount by NHS junior medical staff, both in teaching hospitals and district general hospitals. With the expansion of medical schools this part of the work of consultants is increasing. This work should be fully reflected in the service increment for teaching (SIFT) payments to participating trusts, identified in job plans as a fixed sessional committment, and the necessary adjustments made to the clinical load.

6.4   With the development of multiprofessional and multidisciplinary working, consultants have extended teaching responsibilities to nurses and their other colleagues.

6.5   It is not sufficient that consultants teach: it must be ensured that those who undertake this work are properly trained, both for teaching and assessment of students and trainees.

6.6   Doctors also have a further duty – to ensure that continuing education, research, and good practice are properly valued in their institutions.

ACADEMIC MEDICINE

6.7   Many examples testify to the value of academic medical teaching and research unified with clinical responsibilities.[32] Out of 6343 consultant physicians in 2000,[33] 1036 (16.3%) held academic/NHS appointments, and 73 (1.2%) academic/research appointments.

6.8   Physicians with academic university contracts and honorary NHS consultant appointments make a large contribution to direct patient care in both acute care and the specialties. There are competing demands upon academic physicians and there must be safeguards to ensure that the right balance is maintained between their academic and health service duties. They too must be able to show that they have maintained clinical competence.

RESEARCH

6.9   All modern treatments are a direct result of research. The long-term, continuing improvement in health care depends upon research to yield new means of disease prevention, diagnosis and treatment. Research is also the means of avoiding harm. Research is the only way forward to alleviate and possibly cure distressing conditions that at present cannot be cured.

6.10   Research might include basic research, a contribution to new knowledge on effective health care, oversight of clinical trials, or simply carefully observed changes in practice or the running of a local service. Therefore any consultant might undertake – or encourage or support junior colleagues in undertaking – research of some kind. Naturally, the commitment to research differs between individuals and depends on their skills, interests, priorities, opportunities, the appointments they hold and the institutions they work in. Most physicians have a natural curiosity – honed by training and experience into the critical enquiry that is a necessary element of the clinical consultation – and many have participated in a research study during their studentship and training.

6.11   Many consultants are not in a position to initiate research, secure grants and recruit research staff. They may choose to contribute by participating in collaborative research with better placed academic colleagues, recruiting their patients into clinical trials for example.

6.12   Leadership is as important in research as it is in clinical care; and there is a similar need for appraisal of consultants who undertake this role.

6.13   Doctors have a duty to safeguard the quality of research – its design, conduct and presentation – and always to protect the human subjects of clinical research.[7]

CONSULTANTS IN MANAGEMENT AND ADVISORY ROLES

6.14   Management responsibilities undertaken by consultants include medical directorship, clinical directorship, lead clinician for clinical governance, service review for trust, health authority or the NHS Executive, service planning, clinical tutor, or secretary to a staff committee. Consultants may have formal responsibilities as leaders of clinical teams or their specialist departments.

Medical directors   6.15   NHS trusts are required to appoint a medical director to their board. Medical directors are part of the formal governance arrangements of NHS trusts. They have corporate, professional and management responsibilities, which they may be required to meet by:

- providing professional advice to the trust board and its officers, and coordinating and facilitating the communication of medical professional views on medical matters to the board;
- providing medical input to strategic thinking;
- having management responsibilities for medical staff;
- communicating the trust's perspective to clinicians;
- supporting the work and development of clinical directors;

▓ taking a key role in doctors' disciplinary procedures;

▓ taking part in the management of investigations of a clinical nature concerning doctors, such as those arising from complaints or untoward events; and

▓ taking part in consultant appointment procedures.

Clinical directors 6.16 Many trusts have set up a structure where management responsibility is devolved from the unit to clinical divisions or directorates. A director, who is usually a doctor, leads these. The clinical directors may be charged with:

▓ general management responsibilities;

▓ management responsibilities for other medical staff;

▓ management responsibilities for non-medical staff;

▓ establishing and operating structures for clinical governance;

▓ a range of responsibilities in risk management;

▓ responsibilities in relation to performance and professional self-regulation; and

▓ responsibilities in relation to consultant appointments.

6.17 Sessions need to be allocated in the job plans of consultants who take on the work of clinical director. Doctors with management responsibilities also need to demonstrate their competence in these roles. This will be done with reference to their job plans and the appraisal process.

6.18 Besides these formal management roles, consultant physicians may hold appointments as RCP trust or specialty adviser, or membership of local or multicentre research ethics committees.

6.19 As in their clinical work, doctors in management have a professional duty to ensure that the welfare of patients comes first and must be satisfied that their decisions, advice and actions meet the standards set out in the guidance of the GMC.[34] That guidance also applies to the work of the large numbers of doctors who contribute to the management of health care, lead teams, and have responsibility for the use of resources.

6.20 Policy makers and service managers look to consultants as sources of sound advice. By virtue of their authority and experience, senior consultants are well placed to encourage and participate in local innovation and experiment. Doctors should be familiar with the requirements for effective risk management, particularly in relation to patient care, and be alert to the need for timely advice and action to minimise harm.

Consultants in national roles 6.21 Senior consultants serve in a wide range of activities at the national level, and these command a significant part of their time.[33] They include:

▓ specialist advisory committees (SAC) and training activities;

▓ development and organisation of postgraduate education activities;

▓ clinical governance development and visiting;

▓ National Institute for Clinical Excellence (NICE) guidelines and appraisals;

▓ Commission for Health Improvement (CHI) service inspections;

▓ service on official advisory bodies;

> responses to requests for advice from the Department of Health on information technology, clinical outcomes, national service frameworks;

> support to specialist societies, research funding bodies, charities; and

> the General Medical Council (GMC) and its committees.

6.22   Involvement in management activity is important to the NHS and each role adopted by a consultant should be included within the construct of their job plan. Important roles such as leading a clinical directorate should have a fixed allocation for the task so that there is no clash with clinical duties to the detriment of patients.

6.23   Some activities at national or regional level are just as important to the NHS but do not directly benefit the trust – the immediate employer. Often these appointments are for 2–3 years and should be planned into the work timetable. The contribution of these (often more senior) consultants to regional and national initiatives is vital to the future of the NHS. Guidance from the Department of Health advises trusts that they should be prepared to release staff for such activities.[35]

Recommendations

CONSULTANTS WORKING TO MAINTAIN AND IMPROVE THE QUALITY OF HEALTH CARE
[6.1–6.23]

In addition to patient care the duties and responsibilities of consultants incur other work. Some of this work has an immediate impact upon patient care, but much represents the long-term investment in education and training, academic medicine and research upon which the future safety and quality of heath care, and its advance depends.

The College *recommends* that:

> the time that consultant physicians are required to devote to education and training, academic medicine, research, management and advisory roles – locally and at the national level – should be fully recognised in their conditions of work and in their job plans.

> by precept and example consultants ensure that continuing education, research, and good practice are properly valued in their institutions.

> a consultant's work in each of these areas should be reflected in arrangements for continuing professional development.

7 Consultant workforce

7.1　The most recent annual census of consultant physicians was carried out by the College in September 2000.[33] It asked about working patterns and allocation of time. The findings highlighted issues that are important to the work of the College in setting standards in medical practice and improving the quality of care given to patients.

7.2　There were 6,343 consultant physicians (5,612 whole time equivalents) in the NHS in the UK. Many worked more than the 48 hours specified by the European Working Time Directive. To meet the Directive, at least 1,039 more whole time equivalent (WTE) consultants are required across the UK, mainly in the specialties doing acute general medicine. Were consultants to work only their contracted time, it has been estimated that 3,515 more would be required to maintain the clinical service across the UK.

7.3　Without enough doctors trained as consultant physicians it is not possible to maintain a safe high-quality medical service. The medical specialty bodies have estimated the numbers required to meet the clinical needs of the population; and some have made detailed calculations of the specialist and general medical needs. Overall they show that 100% more consultants are required (see Part 2 of this document).

7.4　Surveys have indicated that most women and some men who currently occupy specialist registrar posts might choose to work part-time. This must be taken into account in planning.

Pattern of consultant work

Direct patient care

i.　Overall, 31% of consultants stated that they were on call for unselected emergency admissions (52% of those who answered the specific question). Specialties most likely to be on call included diabetes and endocrinology, gastroenterology, geriatric medicine and respiratory medicine. Most were on call for patients of all ages, but 29% of geriatricians were only on call for elderly patients. The median frequency of on-call duty was 1:8. 17.5% were on call at more than one location and nearly 20% of consultants were single handed at one of these.

ii.　In the acute medical specialties, 49 patients on average were admitted on take. Physicians in acute specialties transferred an average of 8–13 patients a week to other specialties for particular problems. Over 87% of respondents in these specialties followed up patients with general medical problems in their clinic, an average of 5–9 each week. 7–11 patients admitted each week were not followed up, and 4–7 were transferred to other specialties for outpatient follow-up after discharge.

iii.　Consultants in the acute specialties who undertook general medicine spent an average of 11 hours (range 9–13), mostly in ward work. On average, 3–5 new outpatient referrals each week were general medical.

iv.　Consultants spent an average of 24 hours (range 12–38) per week in their main specialty – on average, 11 hours in outpatients and 7 on the wards. Those in cardiology and gastroenterology spent about 9 hours per week in special procedures.

Pattern of consultant work – continued

Work to maintain and improve the quality of care

v. Consultants have many other responsibilities in the NHS. On average consultants spent a mean of 19 hours (range 10–29) each week in work other than patient care. This generally included education and training, continuing professional development, deanery work, academic and research work, and national work in support of the NHS. Consultants with medical or clinical directorships spent, on average, 5 hours per week on this work.

Recommendations

CONSULTANT WORKFORCE [7.1–7.4]

To maintain a safe, high-quality consultant-led health service in our hospitals, there must be enough consultants to do so. The medical specialties have estimated the numbers of consultants required for the clinical needs of the population. Some have made detailed calculations of the specialist and general medical needs. These calculations show that overall 10% more WTEs are required (see Part 2 of this document).

The College *recommends* that:

■ the consultant workforce be expanded to meet the current and future clinical needs of the population.

■ new ways of providing clinical care be explored to compensate for the shortfall in the consultant workforce.

■ there should be strengthened support and improved facilities to enable consultants to do their work more effectively and more efficiently.

In addition (see Chapter 4), the College *recommends* that:

■ to protect the quality of acute medical care, enough physicians are trained in general internal medicine in addition to a specialty.

Consultants in the medical specialties

WORKFORCE FIGURES [Tables 1–6]

The following tables (pages 27–32) summarise the returns of the 2000 census of consultant physicians. The tables also incorporate estimates of consultant requirements provided by the specialties for Part 2 of this document. These figures may need to be reviewed in the light of recommendations arising out of deliberations that have a bearing on the workforce, such as those on skill mix and National Service Frameworks, besides other developments in practice and service delivery.

Consultants in the medical specialties: numbers in post and estimates of numbers required for UK, England, Wales, Northern Ireland, and Scotland.

Information provided by the medical specialties and from the Royal College of Physicians Consultant Census, September 2000.

Table 1: England, Wales and Northern Ireland. Population 54.7 million (approx).

Specialty	Consultants required* Per 250k population (WTEs)	Consultants required* Total (WTEs)	Consultants in post† (WTEs)	Additional consultants required (WTEs)	Additional consultants required Percentage increase
Audiological medicine	1.25	274	**30**	244	812
Cardiology	5.00	1,094	**556**	538	97
Clinical genetics	0.50	109	**76**	33	44
Clinical neurophysiology	1.10	241	**66**	175	265
Clinical pharmacology and therapeutics	0.70	153	**44**	109	248
Dermatology	3.30	722	**341**	381	112
Endocrinology & diabetes	5.00	1,094	**433**	661	153
Gastroenterology	6.10	1,335	**504**	831	165
Genitourinary medicine	2.10	459	**235**	224	96
Geriatric medicine	6.00	1,313	**773**	540	70
Infectious diseases and tropical medicine	1.00	219	**83**	136	164
Medical oncology	1.25	274	**98**	176	179
Neurology	2.50	547	**289**	258	89
Nuclear medicine	0.85	186	**39**	147	377
Palliative care	1.60	350	**197**	153	78
Rehabilitation medicine	1.80	394	**97**	297	306
Renal medicine	2.10	459	**217**	242	112
Respiratory medicine	5.00	1,094	**451**	643	143
Rheumatology	3.20	700	**352**	348	99
Total	*50*	*11,017*	*4,881*	*6,136*	*126*

* Based on estimates submitted by specialties.
† Figures from RCP Consultant Census 2000.
WTE = whole time equivalent.

NOTES:
1. In developing and/or small specialties the percentage increase is large.
2. For figures for allergy, immunology, intensive care medicine and haematology please refer to the specialty statements.

Table 2: United Kingdom. Population 59.7 million (approx).

| Specialty | Consultants required* | | Consultants in post† (WTEs) | Additional consultants required | |
	Per 250k population (WTEs)	Total (WTEs)		(WTEs)	Percentage increase
Audiological medicine	1.25	299	**31**	268	863
Cardiology	5.00	1,194	**616**	578	94
Clinical genetics	0.50	119	**84**	35	42
Clinical neurophysiology	1.10	263	**72**	191	265
Clinical pharmacology and therapeutics	0.70	167	**55**	112	204
Dermatology	3.30	788	**380**	408	107
Endocrinology & diabetes	5.00	1,194	**489**	705	144
Gastroenterology	6.10	1,457	**555**	902	162
Genitourinary medicine	2.10	501	**249**	252	101
Geriatric medicine	6.00	1,433	**903**	530	59
Infectious diseases and tropical medicine	1.00	239	**101**	138	136
Medical oncology	1.25	300	**112**	188	168
Neurology	2.50	597	**316**	281	89
Nuclear medicine	0.85	203	**47**	156	332
Palliative care	1.60	382	**214**	168	79
Rehabilitation medicine	1.80	430	**113**	317	280
Renal medicine	2.10	501	**255**	246	97
Respiratory medicine	5.00	1,194	**501**	693	138
Rheumatology	3.20	764	**382**	382	100
Total	*50*	*12,025*	*5,475*	*6,550*	*120*

* Based on estimates submitted by specialties.
† Figures from RCP Consultant Census 2000.
WTE = whole time equivalent.

NOTES:
1. In developing and/or small specialties the percentage increase is large.
2. For figures for allergy, immunology, intensive care medicine and haematology please refer to the specialty statements.

Table 3: England. Population 50 million (approx).

Specialty	Consultants required*		Consultants in post[†] (WTEs)	Additional consultants required	
	Per 250k population (WTEs)	Total (WTEs)		(WTEs)	Percentage increase
Audiological medicine	1.25	250	**26**	224	862
Cardiology	5.00	1,000	**500**	500	100
Clinical genetics	0.50	100	**69**	31	45
Clinical neurophysiology	1.10	220	**63**	157	249
Clinical pharmacology and therapeutics	0.70	140	**42**	98	233
Dermatology	3.30	660	**310**	350	113
Endocrinology & diabetes	5.00	1,000	**396**	604	153
Gastroenterology	6.10	1,220	**460**	760	165
Genitourinary medicine	2.10	420	**224**	196	88
Geriatric medicine	6.00	1,200	**696**	504	72
Infectious diseases and tropical medicine	1.00	200	**80**	120	150
Medical oncology	1.25	250	**93**	157	169
Neurology	2.50	500	**277**	223	81
Nuclear medicine	0.85	170	**39**	131	336
Palliative care	1.60	320	**184**	136	74
Rehabilitation medicine	1.80	360	**91**	269	296
Renal medicine	2.10	420	**197**	223	113
Respiratory medicine	5.00	1,000	**411**	589	143
Rheumatology	3.20	640	**329**	311	95
Total	*50*	*10,070*	*4,487*	*5,583*	*124*

* Based on estimates submitted by specialties.
† Figures from RCP Consultant Census 2000.
WTE = whole time equivalent.

NOTES:
1. In developing and/or small specialties the percentage increase is large.
2. For figures for allergy, immunology, intensive care medicine and haematology please refer to the specialty statements.

Table 4: Northern Ireland. Population 1.7 million (approx).

Specialty	Consultants required*		Consultants in post†	Additional consultants required	
	Per 250k population (WTEs)	Total (WTEs)	(WTEs)	(WTEs)	Percentage increase
Audiological medicine	1.25	9	2	7	325
Cardiology	5.00	34	25	9	36
Clinical genetics	0.50	3	1	2	240
Clinical neurophysiology	1.10	7	2	5	274
Clinical pharmacology and therapeutics	0.70	5	1	4	376
Dermatology	3.30	22	12	10	87
Endocrinology & diabetes	5.00	34	13	21	162
Gastroenterology	6.10	41	17	24	144
Genitourinary medicine	2.10	14	3	11	376
Geriatric medicine	6.00	41	26	15	57
Infectious diseases and tropical medicine	1.00	7	1	6	600
Medical oncology	1.25	9	2	7	325
Neurology	2.50	17	5	12	240
Nuclear medicine	0.85	6	0	6	*
Palliative care	1.60	11	7	4	55
Rehabilitation medicine	1.80	12	2	10	512
Renal medicine	2.10	14	9	5	59
Respiratory medicine	5.00	34	12	22	183
Rheumatology	3.20	22	9	13	142
Total	*50*	*342*	*149*	*193*	*130*

* Based on estimates submitted by specialties.
† Figures from RCP Consultant Census 2000.
WTE = whole time equivalent.

NOTES:
1. In developing and/or small specialties the percentage increase is large.
2. For figures for allergy, immunology, intensive care medicine and haematology please refer to the specialty statements.

Table 5: Wales. Population 3 million (approx).

Specialty	Consultants required* Per 250k population (WTEs)	Total (WTEs)	Consultants in post† (WTEs)	Additional consultants required (WTEs)	Percentage increase
Audiological medicine	1.25	15	2	13	650
Cardiology	5.00	60	31	29	94
Clinical genetics	0.50	6	6	0	0
Clinical neurophysiology	1.10	13	1	12	1220
Clinical pharmacology and therapeutics	0.70	8	1	7	740
Dermatology	3.30	40	19	21	108
Endocrinology & diabetes	5.00	60	24	36	150
Gastroenterology	6.10	73	27	46	171
Genitourinary medicine	2.10	25	8	17	215
Geriatric medicine	6.00	72	51	21	41
Infectious diseases and tropical medicine	1.00	12	2	10	500
Medical oncology	1.25	15	3	12	400
Neurology	2.50	30	7	23	329
Nuclear medicine	0.85	10	0	10	*
Palliative care	1.60	19	6	13	220
Rehabilitation medicine	1.80	22	4	18	440
Renal medicine	2.10	25	11	14	129
Respiratory medicine	5.00	60	28	32	114
Rheumatology	3.20	38	14	24	174
Total	*50*	*604*	*245*	*359*	*147*

* Based on estimates submitted by specialties.
† Figures from RCP Consultant Census 2000.
WTE = whole time equivalent.

NOTES:
1. In developing and/or small specialties the percentage increase is large.
2. For figures for allergy, immunology, intensive care medicine and haematology please refer to the specialty statements.

Table 6: Scotland. Population 5 million (approx).
In Scotland, the number of WTEs per head of population is greater than elsewhere in the UK, reflecting geographical and demographic factors.

Specialty	Consultants required*		Consultants in post†	Additional consultants required	
	Per 250k population (WTEs)	Total (WTEs)	(WTEs)	(WTEs)	Percentage increase
Audiological medicine	1.25	25	1	24	2400
Cardiology	5.00	100	60	40	67
Clinical genetics	0.50	10	8	2	25
Clinical neurophysiology	1.10	22	6	16	267
Clinical pharmacology and therapeutics	0.70	14	11	3	27
Dermatology	3.30	66	39	27	69
Endocrinology & diabetes	5.00	100	56	44	79
Gastroenterology	6.10	122	51	71	139
Genitourinary medicine	2.10	42	14	28	200
Geriatric medicine	6.00	120	130	–10	–8
Infectious diseases and tropical medicine	1.00	20	18	2	11
Medical oncology	1.25	25	14	11	79
Neurology	2.50	50	27	23	85
Nuclear medicine	0.85	17	8	9	113
Palliative care	1.60	32	17	15	88
Rehabilitation medicine	1.80	36	16	20	125
Renal medicine	2.10	42	38	4	11
Respiratory medicine	5.00	106	50	50	100
Rheumatology	3.20	64	30	34	113
Total	*50*	*1,007*	*594*	*413*	*70*

* Based on estimates submitted by specialties.
† Figures from RCP Consultant Census 2000.
WTE = whole time equivalent.

NOTES:
1. In developing and/or small specialties the percentage increase is large.
2. For figures for allergy, immunology, intensive care medicine and haematology please refer to the specialty statements.

8 Quality of health care

8.1   In the White Paper, *A first class service*,[36] and many subsequent statements, the Government set out its plans for modernising the NHS and assuring the quality of health care and standards of clinical practice.[37] The features that will have most impact upon the work and practice of clinicians are:

▌ national service standards (National Service Frameworks – NSFs);

▌ promoting clinical and cost effectiveness through guidance and audit (National Institute for Clinical Excellence – NICE);

▌ clinical governance;

▌ reform of professional self-regulation, including revalidation; and

▌ strengthening lifelong learning, of which the chief part is continuing professional development.

CLINICAL GOVERNANCE

8.2   The Department of Health has defined clinical governance as 'the framework through which NHS organisations are accountable for continuously improving the quality of care by creating an environment in which excellence in clinical care will flourish'.

8.3   NHS chief executives are accountable on behalf of trust boards for assuring the quality of NHS trust services. This responsibility is usually delegated to a lead clinician, often a clinical director, who is accountable for ensuring that effective systems of clinical governance are in place.

8.4   Clinical governance confers a responsibility upon individual physicians to work in a way that is consistent with the values and strategic objectives of the organisation that employs them. This enshrines good medical practice. The responsibility of the organisation is to provide appropriate facilities for medical work and to support the professional development of physicians and clinical teams.[38]

8.5   The concept is easily stated, its essence is not new, and its aims are uncontroversial.[39] The vast majority of doctors know and value environments in which excellence flourishes, and they bring their experience and endeavour to make good the shortcomings of those where it does not.

8.6   There is a cost to clinical governance. Besides the cost of administrative structures, doctors implementing the systems may be less available for clinical work. Furthermore, funds diverted to administering the system are not available to repair and develop the infrastructure upon which excellence in practice depends.

MONITORING NHS PERFORMANCE

8.7   The Government has set up a system for assuring and monitoring the performance of the NHS.[36] It comprises:

- Information for Health;
- the National Performance Framework;
- the Commission for Health Improvement (CHI); and
- National Survey of Patient and User Experience.

8.8   The availability of data for these purposes, and their quality, were considered above.

8.9   The components of the Government programme have been usefully summarised in the paper cited.[37] This paper points to opportunities for clinicians to help create the environment for good clinical practice, with the necessary substructure and organisation, and adequate provision for continuing learning and training.

ROLE OF THE COLLEGE IN CLINICAL GOVERNANCE

8.10   The professional bodies have a pivotal role in promoting the highest standards of medical practice. Among the strategic functions of this College are to set and improve standards for clinical practice; to support physicians in their practice of medicine; and to promote and provide continuing professional development throughout a doctor's career.

8.11   The College is well prepared for its role, and has taken action in the following areas towards implementing effective clinical governance.[38]

- a Standards Committee will oversee matters concerning standards of practice;
- the College is collaborating with specialist societies in developing standards for all the specialties represented by the College;
- the Clinical Effectiveness and Evaluation Unit (in close collaboration with the National Institute for Clinical Excellence) will continue the work of producing evidence-based guidelines; act as a clearing house for other relevant guidelines; and develop means of audit;
- the College is working with other Colleges and specialist societies to test systems of team assessment. The College is already piloting schemes involving multidisciplinary assessment and service accreditation;
- the College will further support continuing professional development by investing in the preparation of innovative, interactive CME programmes, and will undertake assessment of CME (CPD) programmes developed by sources other than the College;
- the College will play a key role in setting standards and in maintaining an up-to-date record of continuing professional development and related activities for each consultant;
- the College Standards Committee will seek ways of supporting physicians towards restoring their professional performance;

- the College has a nationwide network of physicians who have specific responsibilities for implementing College policy;
- the College will continue to have a representative function on consultant advisory appointment committees;
- the College will continue to respond to requests from health authorities and trusts to undertake service review;
- the College can provide service support for NHS trusts to help them fulfil their responsibilities for clinical governance; and
- the College has set up the Health Informatics Unit to help make improvements in this area, particularly electronic records in the future.

APPRAISAL

8.12   The new annual appraisal process brings together the discipline of clinical governance, continuing professional development and professional revalidation. The aims of appraisal are to enable NHS employers and consultants to:

- review an individual's work and performance;
- optimise the use of skills and resources to deliver service priorities;
- consider the consultant's contribution to the quality and improvement of services;
- set out personal and professional development needs and agree plans for meeting them;
- identify the resources needed to meet service objectives agreed in the job plan;
- consider support for consultant participation in activities for the wider NHS; and
- utilise the process and associated documentation to meet the requirements for GMC revalidation.

8.13   The content of appraisal will be based on the GMC statement *Good medical practice*,[6] together with relevant management issues, which include the consultant's contribution to the organisation and delivery of local service priorities.[4,40]

PARTNERSHIP WITH TRUST AND HOSPITAL MANAGERS

8.14   To maintain the highest standards of care for patients, clinical teams and trust and hospital managers must work in partnership, being sensitive to each other's responsibilities and to the tensions that these engender.[39] Whilst they must not compromise the standards of their clinical practice, clinicians also have a duty to support managers in meeting their responsibilities to the organisation they all serve.

PRIVATE PRACTICE

8.15   Physicians should apply the same standards of clinical concern to all patients, whether in the NHS or the private sector. They should take care that conduct of their private practice does not compromise NHS duties; and where facilities are shared, the care and investigation of private patients should not be at the expense of patients in the NHS.

Summary points

CLINICAL GOVERNANCE [8.2–8.6]

Clinical governance confers a responsibility upon individual physicians to work in a way that is consistent with the values and strategic objectives of the organisation that employs them. This enshrines good medical practice. The responsibility of the organisation is to provide appropriate facilities for medical work and to support the professional development of physicians and clinical teams.

ROLE OF THE COLLEGE IN CLINICAL GOVERNANCE [8.10–8.11]

The professional bodies have a pivotal role in promoting the highest standards of medical practice. Among the strategic functions of this College are to set and improve standards for clinical practice; to support physicians in their practice of medicine; and to promote and provide continuing professional development throughout a doctor's career.

APPRAISAL [8.12–8.13]

The new annual appraisal process brings together the discipline of clinical governance, continuing professional development and professional revalidation.

PARTNERSHIP WITH TRUST AND HOSPITAL MANAGERS [8.14]

To maintain the highest standards of care for patients, clinical teams and trust and hospital managers must work in partnership, being sensitive to each other's responsibilities.

PRIVATE PRACTICE [8.15]

Physicians should apply the same standards of clinical concern to all patients, whether in the NHS or the private sector.

9 Conclusion

9.1   This statement has described the ways in which consultant physicans meet their duties and responsibilities to serve patients. It also describes the conditions and resources that are necessary to enable patients to have access to medical care of the quality and safety they are right to expect.

9.2   By virtue of the investment in them that society has made, all doctors have a special part in the stewardship of our health care system. The allocation of resources to health care is decided by Government according to its priorities. Insofar as standards of clinical practice and quality of care of patients depend upon the resources made available, individual physicians and the College will continue to seek to influence those decisions.

References

1 Royal College of Physicians. *Consultant physicians working for patients* (1st edn). London: RCP, 1999.

2 Royal College of Physicians. *Consultant physicians responding to change.* London: RCP, 1996.

3 Royal College of Physicians of London. *Hospital doctors under pressure. New roles for the health care workforce. An interim report.* London: RCP, 2000.

4 Central Consultants and Specialists Committee, British Medical Association. *The consultant handbook* (4th edn). London: BMA, 2000.

5 Fletcher CM. Talking with patients: a teaching approach (observations of a Nuffield Working Party on Communications with Patients). London: Nuffield Provincial Hospitals Trust, 1978.

6 General Medical Council. *Good medical practice.* London: GMC, 1998.

7 General Medical Council. *Seeking patients' consent: the ethical considerations.* London: GMC, 1998.

8 Turnberg L. Science, society and the perplexed physician. *J R Coll Physicians Lond* 2000;**34**:569–75.

9 Editorial. A new world of clinical practice. *J R Coll Physicians Lond* 1999;**33**:501.

10 Royal College of Physicians of London. *Management of the older medical patient. Teamwork in the journey of care.* London: RCP, 2000.

11 Kunkler IH. Managed clinical networks, a new paradigm for clinical medicine. *J R Coll Physicians Lond* 2000;**34**:230–3.

12 Anon. Collaborative systematic review of the randomised trials of organised inpatient (stroke unit) care after stroke. Stroke Unit Trialists. *Br Med J* 1997;**314**:1151–9.

13 Editorial. Clinical practice revisited: the importance of the process. *J R Coll Physicians Lond* 2000;**34**:225.

14 Jarman B, Gault S, Alves B, *et al.* Explaining differences in English hospital death rates using routinely collected data. *Br Med J* 1999;**318**:1515–20.

15 Norwell N. The Ten Commandments of record keeping. *Journal of the Medical Defence Union* 1997;**13**:8–9.

16 Rhodes J, Harrison B, Black D, *et al.* General internal medicine and specialty medicine – time to rethink the relationship. *J R Coll Physicians Lond* 1999;**33**:341–7.

17 Royal College of Physicians of London. *Future patterns of care by general and specialist physicians: meeting the needs of adult patients in the UK.* London: RCP, 1996.

18 Federation of Royal Colleges of Physicians of the UK. *Acute medicine: the physician's role. Proposals for the future.* London: RCP, 2000.

19 Royal College of Physicians. *Governance in acute general medicine.* Recommendations from the Committee on General (Internal) Medicine of the Royal College of Physicians. London: RCP, 2000.

20 Royal College of Physicians. *Accident and emergency/acute medicine interface.* London: RCP, in preparation.

21 Mather HM. Coping with pressures in acute medicine. *J R Coll Physicians Lond* 1998;**32**:211–8.

22 Grimley Evans J, Tallis RC. A new beginning for care of elderly people. Editorial. *Br Med J* 2001; **322**:807–8.

23 Department of Health. *Comprehensive initial care: a review of adult initial care services.* London: DoH, 2000.

24 Neale G. Risk management in the care of medical emergencies after referral to hospital. *J R Coll Physicians Lond* 1998;**32**:125–9.

25 McQuillan P, Pilkington S, Allan A, *et al.* Confidential inquiry into quality of care before admission to intensive care. *Br Med J* 1998;**316**:1853–8.

26 Audit Commission. *Setting the record straight: A study of hospital medical records.* London: Audit Commission/HMSO, 1995.

27 Department of Health. NHS Executive Health Services Circular HSC 1998/054. Leeds: NHSE, 1998.

28 Department of Health. *Information for health. An information strategy for the modern NHS.* London: NHSE, 1998.

29 Department of Health. *The NHS performance assessment framework.* London: NHSE, 1999.

30 Dornan TL. The physician as educator. *J R Coll Physicians Lond* 1999;**33**:414–6.

31 General Medical Council. *The doctor as a teacher.* London: GMC, 1999.

32 Editorial. Clinical academic careers. *J R Coll Physicians Lond* 1999;**33**:409.

33 Royal College of Physicians. *Summary of information: consultant workforce in medical specialties in England, Wales and Northern Ireland, 2000.* London: RCP, 2001.

34 General Medical Council. *Management in health care: the role of doctors.* London: GMC, 1999.

35 Department of Health. *Advice to doctors on release of staff for national and regional activities.* Unpublished.

36 Department of Health. *A first class service; quality in the new NHS.* London: DoH, 1998.

37 Cunningham D. Government directives and changes: the potential impact upon clinical practice. *J R Coll Physicians Lond* 1999;**33**:454–7.

38 Royal College of Physicians. *Maintaining good medical practice. Clinical governance and self regulation for physicians.* London: RCP, 1999.

39 Editorial. Clinical governance. *J R Coll Physicians Lond* 1999;**33**:201.

40 General Medical Council. *Revalidating doctors: ensuring standards, securing the future.* A consultation document. London: GMC, 2000.

PART 2

WORK IN THE SPECIALTIES

Introduction

1   Part 1 of *Consultant physicians working for patients* describes the duties and responsibilities of consultant physicians and the ways in which they seek to maintain high standards of patient care. This revised edition brings out more fully the scope and changing conditions of the practice of medicine; and it gives particular attention to acute internal medicine. Part 2 describes each of the specialties of medicine, the work of specialist physicians, and the staff and facilities that are required to carry out this work safely and effectively. It also provides guidance for physicians and managers when they prepare job plans.

SPECIALTY STATEMENTS

2   The specialty committees and societies have drawn up statements, of similar scope, in a common format. We did not wish to stifle accounts of the characteristics of each specialty, or discount variations that are found in practice and delivery of a particular service, and this is reflected in the style and presentation of the statements. But we have sought to ensure that the chief general concerns are brought out in a consistent and balanced way.

3   A chief aim of these statements is to inform and guide the preparation of job plans and the annual appraisal process. They also serve a wider purpose. Each statement has been prepared by responsible bodies of medical opinion, and therefore bears particular authority. They may be referred to as position statements for the specialties.

4   The specialty statements include accounts of:

- The specialty.
- The work of consultants in direct patient care, both in the specialty and in acute medicine, and in work to maintain and improve the quality of care (see paragraph 6).
- Workforce requirements.

5   Broadly, each statement describes:

- The clinical needs of patients that the specialist service seeks to meet.
- Organisation of the service at primary, secondary and tertiary levels.
- Special patterns of referral.
- Ways of working in the specialty, with reference to clinical networks and community arrangements.
- The characteristics of a high quality service, and the requirements for ensuring this, with attention to the clinical workforce, team working, and support staff.
- The clinical work of consultants in the specialty.
- The work of the other members of the multidisciplinary team.
- The chief complementary services that complete the web of care in the specialty. (These are referred to as *conjoined services*, and include nursing services, other specialised clinical services, investigative services, paramedical services, primary care, community services, social services, residential care, hospice care, voluntary services, and non-clinical support).

- The *specialised* facilities required. (The generic facilities and support that every consultant requires are described in Part 1.)
- References to quality standards and measures of the quality of the specialised service, with attention to the chief factors that influence access to service, its safety and quality.
- The contribution made to acute medicine by consultants in the specialty.
- The duties, responsibilities and areas of work of academic physicians, with particular reference to NHS work.
- Developments that offer improved patient care.
- Workforce requirements of the specialty.

6   The work of consultants to maintain and improve the quality of care is protean. It encompasses work in clinical governance, professional self-regulation, continuing professional development, education and training of others, research, serving in management, and providing advice. All these functions require consultant participation, and some clearly fall within the duties and responsibilities of every consultant. Such work is described in detail in Part 1, and is only briefly referred to in the specialty statements. Its scope is set out in Appendix 1, where specific management and advisory work are identified separately.

JOB PLANS

7   The College hopes that consultant physicians will use the specialty statements to inform discussion and negotiation of their job plans with management colleagues. We recommend that each consultant should prepare a job plan with reference to the framework given in Appendix 1. This provides for a job description – the duties and responsibilities of the post – and a work programme. The work programme should seek to quantify both direct patient care and work to maintain and improve the quality of care, together with an account of the resources and facilities required.

Allergy

i   Introduction: a brief description of the specialty and clinical needs of patients

Allergic disorders are wide-ranging and cross the organ-based disciplines. Allergists therefore require expertise specific to allergy and knowledge of areas of a number of other specialities, particularly respiratory medicine, dermatology, ENT and paediatrics. Allergic disease varies from mild to life-threatening. There has been a doubling in prevalence of the commoner allergic disorders, asthma, eczema and rhinitis in the last two to three decades. Superimposed on this there has been a rapid rise in serious allergic disease.

Severe anaphylaxis, originating outside hospitals, occurred in one in 3500 of the UK population per annum in 1994,[1] and the incidence is rising.[2] Anaphylaxis occurs in 1.2 to 16.8% of the US population depending on aetiology.[3] Peanut and nut allergy occurs in over 1% of children;[4,5,6] and latex allergy (second case in 1979) now affects up to 8% of health care workers.[7,8] Others are affected by drug allergy/intolerance and by other food allergies. Much of this serious disease occurs in patients who also have allergic asthma, rhinitis and eczema.

One-third of the population suffer from allergic disease,[9] resulting in considerable direct cost to the health service and impaired quality of life. Allergy is one of the commonest chronic disorders. It has been suggested that part of the increase in prevalence may be related to a westernised life style and lack of infection in childhood.

Traditionally, much of allergy care has been provided by organ-based specialists with an interest, providing a part-time service in allergy, usually in limited areas related to their specialty, or in general practice. The rise in severe and life-threatening allergic disease and multisystem allergic disease has created a new and substantial demand for management requiring the expertise of a consultant allergist. Further, management of the newly emerged disorders (eg nut allergy and latex allergy) requires knowledge gained from dealing with large numbers of patients. This need is largely unmet. It is no longer appropriate for these severe or non-organ based disorders to be dealt with by non-specialists. However there is only a small number of full-time allergists able to provide an appropriate specialist service. Lack of specialist care and long waiting lists for life-threatening disorders are unacceptable.

Before the Calman changes in training, allergy was part of the clinical immunology and allergy training programme, distinct from immunology related to pathology. Training programme changes and delay in allergy going on the Specialist List resulted in uncertainty and an unplanned loss of trainees. The new allergy CCST was recognised in June 1999. Unintentionally, during this interim period there was a reduction in trainee manpower. This is a small specialty, with a need for more consultants and more trainees.

ii   Organisation

Currently allergy services are extremely poor and fail to meet the clinical need.[10] Of 101 allergy services, six are run by consultant allergists providing a full-time service, nine by consultant allergists providing part-time services, and the remaining 86 clinics are part-time and run by organ-based or other consultants who offer a limited spectrum of diagnostic and treatment facilities for allergy. The British Society for Allergy & Clinical Immunology (BSACI) held discussions with the Department of Health (Allergy Task Force) from 1998 to highlight the need and to improve services. This initiative is being taken forward by the National Allergy Strategy Group (NASG) launched at the Royal College of Physicians in May 2001. Current services and proposals for allergy care have been outlined.[11]. There is a shortage of consultant allergists and full-time services lead by consultant allergists are mainly in London and the South-East.

In an ideal model of allergy care there would be four tiers, as follows:[10]

1. the simpler allergic disease would be dealt with in primary care.
2. organ-based and other specialists with an interest (dermatologists, respiratory physicians, ENT specialists, paediatricians, immunologists) would contribute to secondary care.
3. consultant allergists in DGHs and in smaller centres in teaching hospitals would also provide secondary care.
4. Regional allergy centres would deal with the more specialised tertiary problems, and also provide secondary care for their locality. Currently, because of the lack of provision described at 3 above they provide secondary care for a larger area.

There is a lack of provision described at 3 and 4 above, in relation to clinical need, and the majority of general practitioners have little or no training in allergy. The immediate aim is to develop regional allergy centres to provide expertise, improve geographical equality of care and to act as an educational resource and training centre for each region.

Allergy is now a regional specialty and disorders seen in tertiary centres are listed in the Definition of Specialist Allergy Services (London Regional Specialist Commissioning, Definition No 17).

iii Special patterns of referral

Because of the lack of allergists, major centres not only receive tertiary referrals but secondary referrals from outwith their area. There need to be systems to ensure that urgent referrals (anaphylaxis, life-threatening angioedema) are seen quickly. Anaesthetists need rapid access to their regional centre for diagnosis of anaphylaxis during anaesthesia. These networks need to be well established.

iv Ways of working

Allergists should work as part of a team, including specialist allergy nurses. Regional centres should have a minimum of two consultants and ideally 1–2 paediatric allergists; and they need a larger clinical team because of the clinical risks involved in certain procedures (challenge testing) and treatments (immunotherapy). Allergists liaise with other specialists including respiratory physicians, dermatologists, ENT consultants and paediatricians. A clinical immunology laboratory service must be available (run by a consultant immunologist).

There need to be close links with community paediatric teams to provide care for children at risk of anaphylaxis in schools.[12]

Allergists in regional centres have an important role in educating general practitioners, for example, via web sites, and this should reduce referrals.

v   Characteristics of a high quality allergy service

Regional allergy centres should have the following facilities:

Referral

- 24-hour cover and advice from an allergist.
- Review and triage of referral letters.
- Dedicated support staff (secretarial, clerical).
- Standards (determined locally) for time to first appointment for urgent and non-urgent cases. Due to the shortage of allergists this is not 'a reasonable time', but urgent cases should still be seen preferentially.

Outpatient clinics

- Dedicated clinic space, with defined consulting rooms and facilities for day cases.
- Number of patients per clinic. Allergy patients are usually complex, and detailed history taking is essential. A minimum of 45 minutes per new patient is required and 20–25 minutes per follow-up. Four new and one old per clinic, or three new and three old. An immunotherapy clinic would deal with 20–25 patients per 2–3 doctors.
- Specialist allergy nurses.
- Immediate access to treatment for anaphylaxis (this is treated by the allergist). All drugs, IV lines and fluids, oxygen, nebuliser, tilting couches, cardiac arrest box (adult and paediatric).
- Pharmacy service (the supply of drugs for skin testing or challenge; drug information service).
- Dietitians – both adult and paediatric. A dedicated service must be available through the dietetic department. Standard methods of referral to (i) establish if a diet is nutritionally adequate and (ii) provide advice on exclusion diets.
- Full investigations including immunology and imaging.
- Literature: handouts on various disorders eg allergen avoidance; treatment plans for acute allergic reactions; diet sheets; symptom diaries etc.
- Secretarial support. Dedicated staff trained in allergy terminology and policies (allergy practice generates many telephone enquiries from existing and prospective patients).

Day cases

- Facilities for day cases must be available (this may be in outpatients) where patients undergoing challenge tests can remain all day (with appropriate trained nursing staff).
- Challenge tests and immunotherapy are high-risk procedures which must be supervised by a trained consultant.
- Consent forms and information sheets for the above.
- Defined procedures including monitoring for immunotherapy. Accurate record keeping including adverse reactions.

Inpatients

- Access to inpatient beds with junior staff cover.

Patient support groups

- Information should be available and literature displayed.

Communication with GPs

- Letters should be sent to the general practitioner outlining the diagnosis and proposed management.

vi   Outline of clinical work

Most of the work is outpatient or day case based, with only a minimal inpatient component. Most NHS consultants do five clinics a week, some in general allergy and some in specialised clinics according to the consultant's interest; for example, immunotherapy, day case challenge tests; anaphylaxis; venom allergy etc. Diagnostic challenge tests and immunotherapy are an increasing component of the work. In future, novel therapies to replace conventional immunotherapy are likely to increase workload.

Telephone/letter advice is an increasing workload providing advice without seeing the patient. There is also considerable out of clinic work on existing patients, eg patients having further allergic reactions, dealing with schools in the case of children at risk of anaphylaxis; dealing with new acute allergies; updating treatment plans; investigating ingredients of meals; planning/preparing substances for challenge testing.

vii   Work of other members of the multidisciplinary team

Allergy specialist nurses   These are key members of the team. They provide skin prick testing; advice on allergen avoidance; train patients to use self-treatments (adrenaline auto-injectors; inhalers); monitor patients undergoing immunotherapy and challenge tests; support doctors in treatment of acute reactions including anaphylaxis, some using questionnaires to support history taking in defined disorders; and they support follow-up of certain disorders.

Dieticians (adult and paediatric) trained in allergy   Assessment of nutritional adequacy of diet; advice on diagnostic exclusion diets; advice to patients on long term diets. Important role in paediatric allergy.

Pharmacy drug information service   Search for ingredients of drugs; provision of capsules for drugs for challenge tests; information on adverse reactions.

viii   Conjoined services

- Community paediatrician: provision for children at risk of anaphylaxis in his/her area and liaison with colleagues in other health authorities.
- Community paediatric nurses carry out school and nursery visits to train staff in avoidance of allergen (eg nuts), recognition and management of reactions.
- Occupational health. Latex or other occupational allergies; adverse reactions to vaccination.

ix   Specialised facilities

Outpatients and day cases

- Integrated facilities with outpatient and day cases in the same setting improves efficiency and use of expertise.
- A dedicated outpatient area is essential with sufficient couches eg three for safe management of at least 20 patients in one immunotherapy session, in case of anaphylaxis. Sufficient room for resuscitation around each couch is essential.
- Skin testing rooms.

▪ Room(s) for specialist nurse.

▪ Locked refrigerator and drug cupboard storage of therapeutic drugs, vaccines and challenge drugs.

▪ Paediatric play facilities in waiting area and clinic rooms and (ideally) play assistant. Appropriate paediatric dress for nurses and doctors.

▪ Inhalers, nebulisers, oxygen, peak flow meters, spirometry in clinic.

▪ Easy access to lung function laboratory and radiology (close liaison is important).

▪ Equipment for simple ENT examination.

Inpatient facilities

▪ Access to beds, with junior staff cover (many allergy departments share beds and junior staff with the respiratory medicine firm; arrangements should be determined locally).

x   Quality standards

Standards of care need to be defined and developed. There are no national standards, but the BSACI is considering whether regional centres should be accredited.

xi   Contribution to acute medicine

Allergists do not usually participate in the on-call rota for general medicine. Allergy CCST does not certify them in G(I)M. However, consultants in allergy provide:

▪ Consultation service for urgent problems (anaphylaxis, asthma, angioedema, drug reactions).

▪ Consultation service for anaesthetic problems pre-operative or post-reaction

▪ Management of latex allergic patients on elective or emergency admission (in conjunction with Trust Latex Allergy Policy).

▪ Consultation in A&E (eg anaphylaxis).

▪ Urgent training in use of adrenaline auto-injector before discharge from ward or A&E.

xii   Academic allergists

There is a strong tradition of academic allergy in the UK. The NHS workload of academic allergists depends on their academic responsibilities and individual job descriptions. They contribute to the routine work of the NHS Department and often set up tertiary services (specialised clinics). Academic allergists make a major contribution to clinical research. This is essential as in many areas of allergy evidence based guidelines on diagnosis and management need to be developed.

xiii   Developments that offer improved patient care

▪ Referral of patients with nut allergy to specialist allergy clinics (reducing morbidity and mortality by reducing frequency and severity of further reactions, providing effective self-treatment should a reaction occur, reducing A&E attendance and hospital admission, and improving quality of life).[13]

▮ Management of children with glue ear and rhinitis by allergists (recognition of allergic rhinitis as an important cause and treating this means that unnecessary ENT surgery can be avoided).[14,15]

▮ Immunotherapy (efficacy; avoids complications of medical therapy; reduces chronic disease; reduces long term drug use; improves quality of life).[16,17,18]

▮ Challenge testing; likely to improve diagnosis but remains to be evaluated.

▮ Use of specialist nurses: to reduce waiting lists.

▮ Liaison with community paediatricians: to improve care for children at risk of anaphylaxis.[12]

WORK OF CONSULTANT ALLERGISTS

1 Direct patient care

Outpatient work

General allergy clinics

The ratio of new patients to follow-up patients averages 1:2, varying with the complexity of referrals and type of service. The average numbers of patients are three new plus two old patients per doctor. When consultants are training doctors (specialist registrars, GPs, and other consultants) and nurses in outpatient clinics, a consultant can supervise two people per clinic but must allocate extra time to review the patients and teach trainees/students.

An immunotherapy clinic has 20–25 patients.

The number of patients in a day case challenge session depends on the number of doctors and nurses as well as facilities but typically is two patients.

Special clinics within allergy (optional depending on specialist interests and type of centre)

▮ Immunotherapy clinic

▮ Challenge sessions, eg food and drug challenge

▮ Paediatric allergy clinics

▮ Anaphylaxis clinics including nut allergy

▮ Drug and general anaesthetic allergy clinics

▮ Venom allergy clinics

Specialised investigative and therapeutic procedures

▮ Skin prick testing

▮ Immunotherapy

▮ Challenge testing

▮ Occupational allergy testing

All clinics require adequate support staff including specialist nurses. The number of patients seen depends on the complexity of the procedure.

Inpatient work

Referral work: requests for an allergy opinion are common. Ward referrals will be seen on the wards or in outpatient clinics.

There is only a small number of inpatients. Daily ward rounds are required at a minimum as these patients are usually undergoing complex procedures. Rush immunotherapy requires the presence of a doctor at all times during treatment.

On-call

Allergy advice for emergencies and other specialities.

2   Academic medicine

The NHS workload of academic allergists depends on their academic responsibilities and individual job descriptions. They make an important contribution to the work of the NHS Department.

WORKFORCE REQUIREMENTS

At present there are 27 consultant allergists in England (none in Wales, Scotland or Northern Ireland). A review of services by the Scottish Executive recommended creation of allergy posts.[19] Although there are over 100 allergy clinics, most are not run by allergists, but by other specialists with an interest in allergy.[10,20] Many of these clinics were created in response to patient demand. Whilst these consultants make an important contribution to allergy care, this situation fails to comply with clinical governance, and care is inadequate for the increasing number of patients with severe, multi-system or non-organ based allergic disease. There are only six centres with full time allergy services run by allergists (five of which are in London or the Southeast) and nine part-time centres. There are two immediate needs:

1. **To create or staff regional allergy centres (a *minimum* of 1 per region)**
    The National Allergy Strategy Group proposed this as the first initiative, to provide specialist expertise and ensure even geographical distribution.[10,11] This requires a *minimum* of two additional consultants per region* (to reduce long waiting lists, which are 1–2 years in established centres; and to set up services in regions where none exist).

    The numbers of additional consultants required are as follows:

England (8 regions)	16
Wales	2
Total (provision for adult allergy)	18
(including paediatric allergy)	36

2. **To create consultants in DGHs or other teaching hospitals**
    The current provision is so inadequate that even a moderate improvement would require an enormous expansion of consultant numbers.

---

*Note. This does not allow for paediatric allergists (1–2 per region required).

Calculations

Assumptions

Thirty percent of the population have allergic disease. Assume 5/6ths (~85%) will be dealt with in general practice or may not need to see a doctor (possibly 25%). Therefore assume 1/6th of those with allergic diseases (about 5% of the population) need to see a consultant allergist. This figure is based on the prevalence of life-threatening, severe or multi-system allergic disease (see Introduction) ie peanut allergy 1.6%; anaphylaxis up to 16.8%; latex allergy 8% of exposed workers; general anaesthetic anaphylaxis ~1000 cases; other drug allergy/intolerance and other food allergy (incidence not known, but increasing); severe/multi-system allergy, mainly rhino-conjunctivitis, asthma and eczema, up to 5%; immunotherapy 60 cases per million, but 50 attendances per patient; diagnostic challenge tests (numbers not known).

Consultants needed per million population

5% of 1 million = 50,000 patients

1 consultant (7 clinics per week, 4 new + 4 old patients per clinic) will see 1176 new and 1176 old patients p.a. – more if supported by specialist nurses.

5 consultants will see approximately 5,500 new + 5,500 old patients pa.

Thus 5 consultants required per million population (assuming that the at risk population is seen over 10 years). This equates to 1.25 consultants per 250,000 population, therefore 260 consultants are needed for 52 million population (England and Wales).

Present number	27
Additional number for regional centres	18–36 (allowing for paediatrics)
Therefore number required for other centres	215–197

Thus, a total of 233 additional consultants required, a proportion of whom would be in paediatric allergy. This figure could be reduced by, say 20%, as organ-based physicians with an interest in allergy continue to contribute to allergy care.

Trainee manpower

There are few trainees at present. There is a need to increase numbers, otherwise even a minimal consultant expansion is unachievable. This could be achieved incrementally, starting with the six existing major centres. For example:

12 trainees (2 per major centre) would produce 12 consultants in 5 years (24 in 10 yrs); and 20 (2–3 per major centre) would produce 20 in 5 years (40 in 10 yrs).

NOTE: *In 1999 there was insufficient information available to allow a more precise estimate of the workforce requirements in this specialty. This recent estimate provides a firmer basis for workforce planning but this too will need to be reviewed in the light of developments in practice and service delivery.*

References

1. Stewart AG, Ewan PW. The incidence, aetiology and management of anaphylaxis presenting to an accident and emergency department. *Q J Med* 1996;**89**:859–64.

2. Sheikh A, Alves B. Hospital admissions for acute anaphylaxis: time trend study. *BMJ* 2000;**320**:1441.

3. Neugut A, Ghatak AT, Miller RL. Anaphylaxis in the United States: an investigation into its epidemilogy. *Arch Intern Med* 2001:**161**:15–21.

4. Tariq SM, Stevens M, Matthews S *et al.* Cohort study of peanut and tree nut sensitisation by the age of 4 years. *Br Med J* 1996;**313**:514–17.

5. Grundy J, Bateman BJ, Gant C *et al.* Peanut allergy in 3-year old children – a population based study. *J Allergy Clin Immunol* 2001;**107**:S231 (abstract).

6. Chiu L, Sampson HA, Sicherer SH. Estimation of the sensitisation rate to peanut by skin prick test in the general population: results from the National Health and Nutrition Examination Survey 1988–94 (NHANES III). *J Allergy Clin Immunol* 2001;**107**:S192 (abstract).

7. Leung R, Chan HJ, Choy D, Lai CKW. Prevalence of latex allergy in hospital staff in Hong Kong. *Clin Exp Allergy* 1997;**27**:167–74.

8. Liss GM, Sussman GL, Deal K *et al.* Latex allergy: epidemiological study of 1351 hospital workers. *Occup Environ Med* 1997;**54**:335–42.

9. European Allergy White Paper. 1997 Publ. UCB Institute of Allergy, Belgium.

10. Ewan PW. Provision of allergy care for optimal outcome in the UK. *British Medical Bulletin* 2000;**56**:1087–1101 (Ed Kay AB).

11. Ewan PW, Durham SR. *NHS Allergy Services within the United Kingdom: Proposals to improve Allergy Care.* Submitted to *Clinical Medicine.*

12. Vickers DW, Maynard L, Ewan PW. Management of children with potential anaphylactic reactions in the community: a training package and proposal for good practice. *Clin Exp Allergy* 1997;**27**:898–903.

13. Ewan PW, Clark A.T. Long-term prospective observational study of patients with peanut and nut allergy after participation in a management plan. *Lancet* 2001;**351**:111–15.

14. Alles R, Parikh A, Hawk L, *et al.* The prevalence of atopic disorders in children with chronic otitis media with effusion. *Pediatr Allergy Immunol* 2001;**12**:102–6.

15. Parikh A, Alles R, Hawk L, *et al.* Treatment of allergic rhinitis and its impact in children with chronic otitis media with effusion. *J Audiol Med* 2000;**9**:104–117.

16. Varney VA, Gaga M, Frew AJ *et al.* Usefulness of immunotherapy in patients with severe summer hayfever uncontrolled by anti-allergic drugs. *BMJ* 1991;**302**;265–9.

17. Durham SR, Walker SM, Varga E-M *et al.* Long term clinical efficacy of grass-pollen immunotherapy. *N Engl J Med* 1999;**341**:468–75.

18. Nasser SMS, Ewan PW. Depot corticosteroid treatment for hay fever causing avascular necrosis of both hips. *BMJ* 2001;**322**:1589–91.

19. *Immunology and Allergy Services in Scotland,* Scottish Medical and Scientific Advisory Committee, Scottish Executive, 2000.

20. *National Health Service Allergy Clinics* (1998–1999), British Society for Allergy and Clinical Immunology.

Audiological medicine

i Introduction: a brief description of the specialty and clinical needs of patients

Audiological medicine is the medical specialty concerned with the investigation, diagnosis and management of adults and children with disorders of balance, hearing, tinnitus, and auditory communication – including speech and language disorders in children. Approximately 20% of the UK population have significant hearing loss as judged by the MRC National Study of Hearing[1] and one-third of the population experience symptoms of dizziness/imbalance by the age of 60. Despite the prevalence of hearing and balance disorders in the population, the number of consultants in the specialty remains less than the recommended 3/500–600,000.[2]

All patients with audiovestibular needs are right to expect equal and timely access to uniform, good quality care delivered by trained professionals, to prevent or limit impairment disability or handicap. Services should be patient-centred with best practice unrestricted by resources. Children should be given enough time in a child-friendly environment. Patients, their families and carers expect clear, unbiased, up-to-date information in an accessible form. There should be adequate time and expertise for the counselling that is required in chronic disorders and disability. First language interpretation, including sign language, should be available whenever needed, and there should be prompt access to other paramedical and medical disciplines when needed for effective care.

All staff should have adequate time and resources for continuing professional development to ensure that these principles of care are met.

ii Organisation of the service

The specialty is predominantly outpatient based, and provides an audiological, speech and language, and vestibular service. Hospital admission is not normally required, except for a small number of patients with sudden sensorineural hearing loss and/or intractable vertigo and vomiting, and for those who require intensive vestibular rehabilitation. Shared inpatient care with surgical colleagues is required for patients requiring cochlear implantation, bone-anchored hearing aids and vestibular or neuro-otological surgery.

Audiological and vestibular services in the UK remain poorly structured and diverse in organisation. In many NHS Regions the service is unsatisfactory. There is no formal provision of service at primary care level. However, a significant proportion of paediatric audiological services is provided as secondary care in the community, most commonly led by a consultant community paediatrician (audiology). Targeted neonatal and school hearing screening and surveillance are organised as part of the community programme. In some areas this is supervised and supported by a tertiary centre, led by an audiological physician. Sophisticated neuro-otological test facilities, access to cochlear implant programmes, bone-anchored hearing aid programmes and specialised services such as cleft palate clinics are available within departments of audiological medicine. Integrated multidisciplinary care is a key feature of the service.

In other centres, patients who have problems that are are difficult to diagnose, patients who are multiply-handicapped, those with vestibular disorders and other complex problems are referred. Referral is to:

▌ the local ENT Department (in which there may be no specific audiological or vestibular expertise) or

▌ a regional service run by a consultant audiological physician, a consultant otolaryngologist with training in audiology, or a consultant clinical scientist. No second-tier vestibular facilities are available.

In the adult sector, there are no structured audio-vestibular services in primary care. There are some community centres in which adults with hearing impairment may be assessed and provided with auditory amplification. A Royal National Institute for the Deaf (RNID) initiative has promoted the development of direct access hearing aid services for patients over 60 years. These are run by audiologists, working to strict guidelines for referral to an appropriate consultant audiological physician or otolaryngologist.

Audiological physicians provide a tertiary service predominantly in hospital trusts, and in single-handed consultant services that cover the whole spectrum of service provision in audiological medicine, whilst those working in teaching hospitals with other audiological physicians can subspecialise; for example, in paediatric audiological medicine, medical cochlear implantation, speech and language disorders, vestibular medicine or adult auditory rehabilitation. The audiological physician practises general medicine, with particular emphasis on evaluating audio-vestibular function in the context of the overall medical condition. The aetiology of hearing impairment must be determined, appropriate treatment instituted and rehabilitation delivered by a multidisciplinary team. The provision of neuro-otological services for patients with dizziness/vertigo, imbalance or falls is a priority for all departments of audiological medicine. Most departments accept referrals directly from primary care, from second-tier community clinics and at the tertiary level from consultant colleagues.

In order to be most effective, each department of audiological medicine should serve a population of approximately 500,000, ideally with three but no less than two whole-time equivalent consultants in audiological medicine spanning all aspects of the specialty.

iii Special patterns of referral

In paediatric practice, referrals derive from general practitioners, failures of screening programmes; and from community paediatricians for the evaluation of complex auditory disorders, vestibular disorders, the multiple-handicapped child and speech and language-disordered children. Paediatric referrals are also received at the tertiary level, primarily from otolaryngologists, paediatricians and geneticists.

In adult practice, patients are most commonly referred by general practitioners and at the tertiary level from otolaryngology, neurology, geriatrics and psychological medicine.

iv   Ways of working, clinical networks and community arrangements

Audiological medicine depends upon a multidisciplinary team including audiologists, speech and language therapists, hearing therapists, educational audiologists, hearing aid audiologists, psychologists and physiotherapists to ensure both accurate diagnosis and optimal rehabilitation.

The audiological physician should provide guidance, teaching and supervision of the range of screening programmes for hearing loss in children, the initial assessment of children in primary centres, and assessment in secondary/community centres for hearing, communication and development should be in place. A full clinical service should be provided in tertiary centres for audiovestibular disorders and complex communication disorders. There should be access to all medical disciplines relevant to the investigation of the aetiology of hearing and balance disorders, with access to sophisticated audiological and vestibular test equipment.

The audiological physician provides a counselling and information service for parents of newly diagnosed deaf children and is pivotal in enrolling the multidisciplinary team to ensure early communication specialists for preschool intervention, access to the deaf children/adult role model/mentor and access to sign-supported English. Educational and psychological assessments are required and there must be long-term multidisciplinary support to ensure optimal intellectual, social and personal development of each child, and a seamless transfer to adult care.

In adult practice, the audiological physician will similarly coordinate and be supported by a multidisciplinary team comprised of a psychologist, hearing therapist, audiologists, physiotherapists and speech and language therapists, to ensure not only accurate diagnosis and medical treatment, but appropriate rehabilitation for the hearing impaired adult.

The audiological physician will investigate and manage tinnitus, and have adequate training in neurology and paediatrics to provide a specialist vestibular service for both children and adults.

v   Characteristics of a high quality service

A high-quality service depends upon the integration of audiological medicine into the national provision of otological services. Three consultants in audiological medicine should practise with four ENT surgeons, three to four doctors, at SHO/SpR level, two audiological scientists, one MT05, four MTO4, two MTO3 and four ATO audiologists, two speech and language therapists for the hearing impaired, two educational audiologists, one deaf role model/sign language teacher, a social worker/counsellor, two medical secretaries, three receptionists, and two records clerks.

This multidisciplinary team will meet the quality standards for the detection of children with significant hearing loss as proposed by the National Deaf Children's Society,[3] and ensure all services are child- and family-centred. Written policies on availability of first-language interpreters including British Sign Language. Speech and language therapists for all hearing-impaired children would be available. A full range of hearing aids would be available, allowing one spare instrument per child. These would be prescribed on a 'right-first-time ' basis, which is likely to require pre-programmable aids from the outset. All equipment and facilities would conform to a minimum standard, and national guidelines on waiting times would be met. All aspects of the service would be audited.

In the paediatric domain, all hearing-impaired children would be identified before four months of age, all hearing-impaired children would have access to appropriate amplification, educational support, and aetiological investigation.

A multidisciplinary assessment would ensure appropriate provision of oral and/or aural communication training and integrated care across health, education and social services, to promote optimal physical, emotional and mental health. A high-quality service would ensure a seamless transition from paediatric to adult care with appropriate psychological support if required during adolescence.

In adult practice, all patients with auditory symptoms, including hearing loss, tinnitus and dysacuses would have rapid access to diagnostic and rehabilitation facilities. All hearing aids should be provided on a 'right-first-time' basis and a full range of hearing aids should be available. Sudden hearing loss is a medical emergency and provision for admission, investigation and appropriate management is essential.

A multidisciplinary team would ensure joint rehabilitative care with social services, to optimise both occupational opportunities and domestic needs.

A high-quality service in audiological medicine would ensure provision of eye movement assessment and vestibular and balance assessments in patients with symptoms of dizziness, vertigo, falls and ataxia. Prompt investigation together with multidisciplinary rehabilitation are essential, with particular input from otolaryngology, neurology, psychiatry and physiotherapy.

vi   Clinical work of consultants in the specialty

Consultants in audiological medicine provide an inpatient service across many disciplines including paediatrics, neurology, oncology, ophthalmology, cardiology, general medicine, otolaryngology, geriatrics, genetics and psychiatry, to provide an opinion on auditory and vestibular function in the context of the overall medical diagnosis of a patient. Most inpatients are seen in the outpatient department where appropriate audio-vestibular test facilities are available; but critically ill patients are assessed on the ward, or in the intensive care unit, for therapeutic advice until they are well enough to be brought to the outpatient department for detailed testing.

The primary workload is in providing an adult and paediatric outpatient service, supervising the diagnosis, management strategy and rehabilitation service for patients with hearing and balance disorders.

vii   Work of other members of the multidisciplinary team

The multidisciplinary team includes:

▌ *Audiologists (audiology technicians)* who are responsible for equipment calibration, routine audiometric and vestibular testing of patients, the provision and simple repairs of hearing aid systems.

▌ *Audiological scientists* are responsible for the maintenance and calibration of equipment, the development of test protocols and new testing techniques, the site of lesion investigation of complex auditory and vestibular disorders, and the development of appropriate management strategies and outcome measures. They are involved in research and audit, teaching and clinical developments.

▌ *Speech and language therapists* define speech and language disorders, and support the development of communication skills, advising on appropriate therapy.

▌ *Hearing therapists* support the hearing-impaired, advising on hearing tactics, provide counselling with regard to negative percepts of hearing loss and tinnitus, and participate in the overall rehabilitation strategy.

▌ *Psychologists/behavioural therapists* are crucial in the rehabilitation process in both hearing and balance disorders which are associated with significant psychological symptoms and disorders.

▌ *Educational audiologists* play a major role in integrating deaf children into the normal educational system and supporting children to maximise their potential in hearing-impaired units of mainstream or special schools.

▌ *Physiotherapists* are key members of the vestibular rehabilitation team, constructing customised vestibular exercises, instructing patients on gait strategies and ensuring appropriate musculo-skeletal function to enable good balance.

viii Conjoined services

Conjoined services include nurses in tertiary centres and health visitors in the community, together with scientists, therapists and psychologists in hospital centres. Other clinical disciplines include otolaryngology, neurology, geriatrics, psychiatry, paediatrics, genetics, and cardiology. Investigative services include haematology, clinical chemistry, microbiology, radiology and electrophysiology. Social services are important in terms of both employment and appropriate domestic support. Voluntary bodies, including RNID and NDCS, play a very significant role in ensuring appropriate facilities for the hearing impaired and laying down criteria for good practice, and the deaf community is particularly important in providing support.

ix Specialised facilities

Suitable space is required for the provision of auditory and vestibular testing. All rooms must meet health and safety requirements and be suitable for infection control. All facilities should have pushchair and wheelchair access and audiometric booths must meet international standards.

Specialised facilities required by an audiological medicine service

Hearing testing:

Paediatric
    3 large paediatric sound-proof test booths with viewing areas
    1 standard booth with viewing area for children
    1 child-friendly hearing aid fitting room
    1 acoustically-treated child-friendly hearing aid prescription room
    1 parent counselling room

Adult
    4 standard audiometric sound-proof test booths
    1 evoked-response booth
    2 acoustically-treated hearing aid prescription rooms
    3 hearing aid fitting rooms
    2 comfortable rooms for hearing therapy
    1 large room for group relaxation classes
    seminar room
    waiting room
    5 offices for 2 people each

continued

Vestibular testing:

Paediatric
   A child-friendly, purpose-designed, dark vestibular test room with play area
Adult
   2 large, dark vestibular laboratories with sink and clean mains water
   A large room for group relaxation and balance retraining
   Counselling and cognitive therapy room.

Specialised facilities include a full range of sophisticated audiological test equipment (audiometers, visual-reinforced audiometry, impedance bridge, otoacoustic emission equipment, speech audiometry, electro-physiological equipment and central auditory test facilities) together with appropriate resources and facilities for calibration of all equipment, and prescription of hearing aids.

Specialised vestibular equipment includes facilities for caloric testing, eye movement recording including electro-oculography and/or video-nystagmography, and, in specialised centres, rotational testing and posturography. Access to tertiary radiology (with provision for MRI/CT with anaesthesia) genetics, neurological, otological, ophthalmological and paediatric facilities are essential for diagnosis and access to psychological, physiotherapy and speech and language therapy is essential for rehabilitation.

The up-to-date equipment (less than 5 years old) required for a population of 500,00 includes a facility for universal neonatal screening and digital hearing aid provision is given below. Such equipment is required for at least six sites across hospital and community. (See draft document *Audiological medicine in a modern NHS*, British Association of Audiological Physicians, 2001.2)

Recommended equipment (<5 years old) for a population of 500,000

Hearing testing equipment:

Paediatric
   4 otoacoustic emissions systems (+ 2 for screening)
   2 auditory brainstem evoked response systems
   5 sets of distraction test equipment
   3 sets for visual reinforcement audiometry
   5 sets of toy test material for speech audiometry
   2 children's wordlists on tape
   5 hand held sound field audiometers
   5 sound level meters
   6 clinical audiometers with insert earphones, conventional earphones, and speaker outlet
   Bekesy/audioscan for testing failures
   4 hearing aid test boxes with real ear measurement and prescription programming.
   4 tympanometers
   8 otoscopes
   3 head lights for direct vision
   2 operating microscopes for aural toilet
   10 probes, etc. for wax removal
   2 sets of equipment for syringing wax
   video-otoscope
   2 ultrasonic cleaners

continued over

Adult

3 clinical audiometers	2 otoacoustic emissions systems
2 tympanometers	3 real ear measurement systems
2 tape recorders for speech testing	3 environmental aids displays
2 sound field systems	1 minicom telephone
2 brainstem evoked response systems	3 ultrasonic cleaners
comfortable relaxing chairs	3 earmould grinders

Vestibular testing equipment:

rotating chair + computerised programme	electro-oculography
2 videonystagmoscopes	2 reclining couches with
access steps	
2 bithermal caloric irrigators	2 Barany drums
dynamic posturography	1 full field optokinetic system
2 Frenzel's glasses	2 laser lights for eye movement stimuli
	1 infrared viewing system

x   Quality standards

The document *Audiological Medicine in a modern NHS*, published in 2001[2] by the British Association of Audiological Physicians, sets out the standards to be expected in a high-quality service. The National Deaf Children's Society has laid down quality standards for the care of children with hearing loss,[3] and the Royal National Institute for the Deaf has drawn attention to inadequacies in the current provision of audiological services nationwide. Auditory and vestibular disability/handicap questionnaires are widely used to evaluate outcome of auditory and vestibular intervention in clinical practice.

The chief factors limiting appropriate access to service include inadequate numbers of audiological physicians, audiologists and support staff – and inadequate training. There is also limited awareness, both within the profession and the lay public. Absence of appropriate specialised departments results in patients being seen in a variety of different disciplines, which perpetuates a fragmented, poorly resourced and inadequately structured service.

xi   Contribution to acute medicine

Consultants and SpRs in audiological medicine do not participate in the on-call rota for acute general medicine. They do, however, manage two acute presentations: sudden hearing loss and acute intractable vertigo. Both conditions require urgent admission, investigation and management.

xii   Academic audiological medicine

Audiological Medicine is a developing specialty, with only three professors and three academic trainees.

The academic staff have taken a lead in training, research, and piloting and validating new rehabilitation and management strategies. They are responsible for taking the lead in promoting evidence-based medicine and supporting clinical governance throughout the specialty. Each academic department runs a tertiary clinical service: paediatric audiological medicine (Manchester), adult auditory rehabilitation (Cardiff), and vestibular medicine (London).

Two of the units run MSc programmes in audiological medicine, one in London and one in Manchester, as part of the higher specialist training programme in this specialty.

xiii Developments that offer improved patient care

Current proposals and developments to improve the provision of audiological care include:

- *Universal neonatal screening* is a recent initiative with pilot sites currently evaluating the efficacy and feasibility in the UK, using otoacoustic emissions. A critical review[4] has clearly demonstrated that universal neonatal hearing screening is the most cost-effective and highest-yield method of defining congenital bilateral hearing impairment. The introduction of this programme is currently limited because of inadequate resources, but allocation of resources and service as outlined above would facilitate appropriate expansion.

- *Direct access clinics* for the provision of auditory care to the over-60s is currently offered by a number of trusts but also requires expansion and the development of clear guidelines for medical referral.

- *One-stop vestibular clinics* for the dizzy patient are required to limit the occupational and social morbidity caused by disorders of balance.

- The current government initiative, termed *'Action in ENT'* programme, which includes audiological medicine, is piloting a variety of local and national projects to improve access to patient care.

- The introduction of *digital hearing aids* into the NHS is currently being piloted nationwide.

WORK OF CONSULTANTS IN AUDIOLOGICAL MEDICINE

1 Direct patient care

A Work in the specialty

Inpatient work

Audiological medicine provides a service to inpatients in paediatrics, neurology, oncology, ophthalmology, cardiology, general medicine, otolaryngology, geriatrics, genetics and psychiatry, providing an opinion on auditory and vestibular function in the context of the overall medical diagnosis of a patient, eg:

- audiovestibular problems in relationship to ototoxicity and radiotherapy,

- auditory and vestibular site of lesion diagnosis in neurological, genetic and paediatric disorders,

- management and rehabilitation of auditory and vestibular sequelae of general medical/paediatric disorders.

In a district general hospital, two such cases may be seen in each outpatient clinic. In a busy teaching hospital a separate session should be allocated twice a week for evaluation of inpatient referrals. Up to six such patients could be seen in one session.

In teaching hospitals, audiological medicine forms part of the postgraduate teaching programme, including grand rounds and case conferences.

Outpatient work

The consultant audiological physician, working alone in an adult outpatient clinic, may see 4–6 new patients and 4–8 follow-up patients in a session. The number will depend on the consultant's experience, the complexity of the problem and the availability of support staff. Whenever possible, audiovestibular investigations should be carried out at the same attendance. In a paediatric clinic, up to six patients in total may be seen, the precise number depending on the type of clinic.

Specialist clinics include tinnitus, dizziness, cleft palate, bone-anchored hearing aid, cochlear implantation and neonatal screening clinics. A single-handed consultant could undertake no more than one such clinic each week.

Outpatient review of inpatients   Review of inpatients under the care of other specialties varies depending upon the nature of the hospital but 0.5 NHD a week should be allocated for this activity in a DGH and up to 1.0 NHD in teaching hospitals.

Outpatient activities   The diagnostic and rehabilitative, auditory and vestibular, and paediatric and adult workload varies between centres. The clinical work should be divided equally between adults and paediatric, but clinics should be held separately to ensure child-friendly environments. All clinics should provide full medical diagnostic and therapeutic approaches to auditory and vestibular disorders and there should be appropriate access to general medical and paediatric outpatient services.

Specialised investigative and therapeutic procedure clinics

Specialised clinics within audiological medicine vary considerably from trust to trust, depending on the nature of the hospital, the allocation of resources, the workload of the individual consultant and the availability of support from other medical disciplines. The aim of all clinics should be to provide a 'one-stop' service.

Electrophysiological testing   Complex electrophysiological testing such as middle ear latency responses, cortical-evoked responses and brainstem-evoked responses in children, particularly if requiring anaesthesia, may be conducted in separate specialised clinics of 2–4 patients. The number of such clinics will depend on the caseload of each individual consultant, varying between one a week and one a month.

Vestibular test clinics   In some centres, due to lack of resources, vestibular investigations are undertaken at a separate attendance. Depending on the age of the patient, the complexity of the testing and the resources, three to six patients may be tested in one weekly session.

Central auditory testing   The complexity and time-consuming nature of central auditory testing requires the provision of separate test time; 2–4 patients may be tested in one session.

Hearing aid assessment clinics   Specialised therapeutic procedures clinics may be required for the provision of hearing aids in complex cases to allow evaluation of the patient's needs, matching of the instrument, and modifications of the sound-delivery system.

Specialised services within the specialty

The specialised clinics provided within a department of audiological medicine depends on the setting – whether it is a district general hospital or a teaching hospital, the number of consultants in audiological medicine working in one unit, the support of other medical disciplines, particularly otolaryngology, and the workload feasible within the limitation of available resources.

Supervision of rehabilitation service This service is run on a day-to-day basis by members of the multidisciplinary team, and includes the provision, servicing and modification of hearing aids, bone-anchored aids, cochlear implants and environmental aids. In addition, the audiological physician may oversee the direct-access clinics for the provision of hearing aids to the over 60-year-old patient. At least one NHD a week should be allocated for this task.

Adult vestibular service One NHD should be allocated for providing a 'dizzy' clinic, which typically requires more doctor time per patient than a routine adult hearing clinic. Adequately skilled technical and scientific staff are required if investigations are to be efficiently conducted in a 'one-stop' format and access to support and conjoined services outlined above is required.

Adult tinnitus clinics Fewer patients are seen per clinic than in a routine 'hearing' clinic and the service is best provided in a multidisciplinary framework. One NHD a week should be allocated and supported by a clinical psychologist and at least one hearing therapist.

Adult learning disability hearing clinic This service requires the multidisciplinary facilities of the paediatric audiological medicine clinic; 0.5 NHD per week should be allocated. Patients with mental health problems are also best seen in this setting.

Paediatric clinics Two NHDs a week should be allocated for a multidisciplinary paediatric audiological medicine clinic. Ancillary staff must include a hearing therapist, speech and language therapist, advisory teacher for the hearing impaired, educational psychologist, audiological technicians and audiological scientists. There must be access to paediatrics, clinical genetics, neurology and otolaryngology.

Supervision of screening and surveillance programmes Audiological physicians commonly oversee neonatal and school screening and surveillance programmes together with the ongoing rehabilitation needs of those with hearing impairment. One NHD per week is required to evaluate children who fail the neonatal screen, requiring detailed investigation, sophisticated rehabilitative techniques and adequate time for parental discussion. With the current government initiative to introduce a universal neonatal screening programme nationwide, this workload will increase.

Paediatric vestibular service 0.5 NHD should be allocated to the provision of this service. It requires the same facilities as the adult service, in a child-friendly environment.

Teaching sessions Fewer patients can be seen at these sessions in which training of junior medical staff and paramedical staff is being undertaken.

Services outwith the base hospital

The present numbers of audiological physicians preclude the provision of a high-quality service nationwide. Therefore many audiological physicians undertake clinics in more than one hospital or as outreach clinics in District General Hospitals, community clinics and in primary care groups. The scope of this work and the way in which the clinics are conducted varies widely.

For those unable to attend hospital clinics for the provision of hearing aids and appropriate auditory rehabilitation, domiciliary visits or visits to old peoples' homes are arranged; and there are visits to schools for the deaf and hearing-impaired units to provide support for hearing-impaired children.

On-call advice for emergencies

There is no formal on-call requirement for consultants in audiological medicine.

WORK PROGRAMME OF A CONSULTANT IN AUDIOLOGICAL MEDICINE

Example of the work programme of a consultant physician in audiological medicine.

1 Direct patient care

Activity	Workload	NHDs allocated per week	Clinical support	Conjoined services
Work in the specialty				
Inpatient work	4–8 patients	0.5–1.0	Full audiological and vestibular multidisciplinary team as above	As listed above for adult/ paediatric provision
Specialised services	Outpatient clinics[1] (include investigative & therapeutic procedures – Maximum 6 therapeutic procedures)	0.5		
	New patients (4–8 adult patients per clinic; up to 6 children)			
	Follow-up patients (4–12 adult patients per clinic; up to 6 children)			
	Outpatient review of inpatients (4–12 adult patients per clinic; up to 6 children)			
	Adult audiological diagnostic and rehabilitation service			
	Adult vestibular service			
	Adult tinnitus clinics			
	(Maximum 4 electrocochleograms and/or auditory brainstem responses (ABRs) for paediatric diagnosis, in a session) (4–8 patients per clinic)			
	Adult learning disability hearing clinic	2		
	Paediatric clinics	1		
	Neonatal hearing service	0.5		
Work outside the base hospital	Paediatric vestibular service	1–2		
On-call for specialist advice and emergencies	Depends on available resources Depends on the centre	} 0.1–1		

continued

Acute medicine	Very rare	0.1	N/A	N/A
On-take	None	0	N/A	N/A
Academic medicine	Approx. 1/3 clinical	4	As for consultant	As for consultant
	Approx. 1/3 teaching	3–4		
	Approx. 1/3 research	3–4		

¹ Normally fixed each week. Formal teaching is normally at fixed times.

2 Work to maintain and improve the quality of care*

Encompasses work in clinical governance, professional self-regulation, continuing professional development, education and training of others, research, serving in management, and providing advice. All these functions require consultant participation, and some clearly fall within the duties and responsibilities of every consultant.

Total time allocated to these activities   *2–4 NHDs*

A 50–50 split between paediatric and adult outpatient clinics is assumed for the purposes of the above table, although the distribution of work varies widely for individual jobs and individual trusts.
*See Appendix to Part 2 of this document for a detailed breakdown.

The total number of sessions worked and their distribution varies between consultants. Most work programmes indicated an excess of ten units worked. There are times in the career of a consultant when management and national duties increase the number of sessions.

WORKFORCE REQUIREMENTS FOR AUDIOLOGICAL MEDICINE

The document *Audiological medicine in a modern NHS* ² contains recommendations for the staff required to serve a population of 500,000. This includes vestibular and hearing services combined – for children and adults – in community and hospital sites, allowing for universal neonatal hearing screening and digital hearing aid provision, and ensuring that each professional has a peer. It refers also to the staff required for a team based at main unit working across several sites and providing support for ENT clinics.

A minimum of three whole-time equivalent consultant audiological physicians, one consultant community paediatrician (audiology) and one whole-time equivalent consultant audiological scientist (state registered audiologist) is required for a population of 500,000–600,000, with appropriate junior medical staff and a multidisciplinary team of audiological staff.

Each trust should have a purpose-designed audiological centre in which an appropriate number of consultant physicians and other staff are based, and from which primary care and community-based services can be delivered, monitored and developed on an integrated multiple hub-and-spoke model. The activity of a department of audiological medicine is most effective when integrated with a department of otolaryngology.

Audiological centres must include a multidisciplinary team with specialist speech and language therapists for the hearing impaired, hearing therapists, audiological scientists, audiologists, educational audiologists, physiotherapists, psychologists, nursing staff, and adequate administrative staff comprised of secretaries, receptionists and A and C records staff.

NOTE: *In 1999 there was insufficient information available to allow a more precise estimate of the workforce requirements in this specialty. This recent estimate provides a firmer basis for workforce planning but this too will need to be reviewed in the light of developments in practice and service delivery.*

Staffing requirement for the service provided by an audiological centre

Professional		Child		Adult	Total
Audiological physician (Consultants in ENT)		1		1 (+1)	3
Non-consultant career grade, SHO and SpR		2		2	4
Audiological scientists	Grade C	1	or	1	1
	Grade B	1	or	1	1
	Grade A	1	or	1	1
Audiologist	MTO5	1		(1)	1–2
	MTO4	2		2	4
	MTO3	1		1	2
	MTO2	1		1	2
	MTO1	0		2	2
	ATO	2		2	4
SALT for hearing impaired		2		1	3
Educational audiologists/ATHI		2		0	2
Deaf role model/sign language teacher		1		0	1
Social worker/counsellor		1		1	2
Hearing therapist		0		2	2
Physiotherapist		0		1	1
Psychologist		1		1	2
Nurse/health care assistant		1		3	4
Medical secretary		2		2	4
Receptionists		2		2	4
A and C records staff		2		2	4

References

1. Davis, AC. *Hearing in adults.* London: Whurr, 1995.

2. *Audiological medicine in a modern NHS.* London: British Association of Audiological Physicians, 2001.

3. National Deaf Childrens Society. *Quality standards in Paediatric Audiology.* Vol. 1, 1994; Vol. 2, 1996. London: NDCS.

4. Bamford J, Davis A. Neonatal hearing screening: a step towards better services for children and families. *Br J Audiol* 1998;**32**:1–6.

Cardiology

i Introduction: a brief description of the specialty and clinical needs of patients

Cardiology encompasses all aspects of the care of patients with heart disease. Paediatric Cardiologists deal with heart disease in babies and children up to adolescence, and collaborate with adult cardiologists in dealing with congenital heart disease in adolescent and grown-up patients (GUCH – grown-up congenital heart disease). This specialty statement deals specifically with adult cardiology, in which many consultants also practise general medicine.

Coronary heart disease (CHD) remains the commonest cause of death in the UK. Despite huge advances in diagnosis and treatment over the last decade, the provision of care for patients with heart disease has not kept up with the increased demand that these advances have created.[1]

The specialist service seeks to meet the need for comprehensive risk assessment and risk modification, involving medical treatment of symptoms, investigation of symptoms to define risk, and for treatment of symptoms and disease by drugs, non-surgical intervention or surgery as appropriate. Cardiac rehabilitation and secondary prevention are usually established by specialist care. The service is also involved in palliation of conditions which are not at the present time amenable to cure. These requirements for CHD patients are reflected in the National Service Framework for CHD.[2]

ii Organisation of the service at primary, secondary and tertiary levels

The service is becoming highly integrated between these three levels of care. The aim is to provide a seamless transition for the patient from primary to secondary and then to tertiary care as necessary and back within cardiac networks based on a tertiary centre operating to agreed protocols.[2]

The main emphasis in *primary care* is in the prevention of disease, the assessment of risk and the maintenance of a coronary artery disease register. In addition, in primary care the symptoms of the disease must be recognised, correctly diagnosed and correct treatment started. Many of these patients will need to be referred on to secondary care for further assessment and treatment. Primary care also has an important role in maintaining rehabilitation and secondary prevention.

In *secondary care* patients are further diagnosed and investigation undertaken. This ranges from reassurance for minor but important complaints to emergency lifesaving treatment for patients with myocardial infarction. It is particularly important that treatment is delivered quickly when necessary. In particular, re-establishing coronary flow in patients sustaining heart attacks is of high priority in most secondary and tertiary care. In secondary care investigations such as coronary angiography are also carried out. If patients require interventions such as angioplasty or coronary artery bypass surgery they are generally referred for tertiary care, although certain forms of intervention (but not surgery) are becoming possible in secondary care.

Tertiary care delivers very specialised investigation and treatment. This includes most aspects of electrophysiology and intervention for coronary artery disease. In addition, cardiac surgery is carried out exclusively in tertiary centres. There are some forms of treatment that should be classified as being more specialised than that provided by the average tertiary centre. These include cardiac transplantation and the management of pulmonary hypertension. These are under the control of NSCAG. Services for adolescents and grown-ups with congenital heart disease are provided mainly in the tertiary centre in so-called GUCH clinics.

iii Special patterns for referral

The normal pattern of referral is via the general practitioner to either the secondary or tertiary centre. The exception is that referral for cardiac surgery is restricted to cardiologists. Cardiac surgeons do not accept direct referrals from primary care physicians or consultant general physicians.

Urgent referrals – patients with suspected recent onset of angina should be seen within 2 weeks in rapid access chest pain clinics currently being set up following the National Service Framework.

Patients with acute coronary syndrome should be admitted and referred urgently to a cardiologist. A significant number of these patients will require early angiography and revascularisation.

iv Ways of working, clinical networks and community arrangements

Networks of care are being developed all around the country. The aim is to produce a seamless pattern of care for the patient from the first point of contact with the healthcare system to whatever complex investigation or treatment is required. These networks of care are being set up by collaboration between primary, secondary and tertiary care, and are based on a tertiary centre and its catchment.[2]

Cardiologists lead multidisciplinary teams within secondary and tertiary care. These involve particularly cardiac nurses and technicians but expanding in quality and practice development teams to include rehabilitation and prevention professionals, and other relevant hospital departments, eg A&E, so that whole clinical pathways are represented. Primary care should become more involved in these as many districts are developing primary/secondary care interface services with rapid access for non-invasive assessment. As local implementation teams for the NSF have developed therefrom, community prevention agencies have been involved alongside management.

Clinical care pathways, defined by protocols in place from 1 April 2001, are now ripe for audit, eg the Myocardial Infarction National Audit Project (MINAP)[4] now in place for acute myocardial infarction (Clinical Effectiveness and Evaluation Unit, Royal College of Physicians).

v Characteristics of a high quality cardiology service

The criteria of the high quality service are as follows:
- It is appropriate and responsive to patient need.
- There is sound quality assurance, maintained by audit and clinical governance.
- Communication with the patient is kept at the forefront and is extremely important.

▪ This care can only be delivered by an integrated team comprising nurses, technicians and doctors. These clinical workers are backed up by service managers. They are essential in providing the wherewithal with which to provide the service.

▪ It also essential that there is adequate backup from IT and secretarial services. Indeed, good secretarial services are the linchpin of a good clinical service.

The Fifth Joint Report on Cardiothoracic Services[1] will develop a detailed analysis of service requirements. The National Service Framework for CHD[2] enumerates 12 standards of care (see x below).

vi Quality standards and measures of the quality of the specialised service

The National Service Framework for CHD[2] has emphasized the inequalities that exist in access to service; social, geographic, ethnic, gender and age factors being important as well as variation in the quality of provision of service. Twelve standards of care have been developed for networks to implement with dated milestones for achievement of protocols, registers and audit data, and performance indicators. The Myocardial Infarction National Audit Project (MINAP) database[4] will capture many of the clinical secondary care data required to prove quality of service.

vii Developments that offer improved patient care

▪ Co-ordination of primary care with secondary and tertiary care to deliver cardiac care particularly in prevention

▪ Two week wait rapid access chest pain clinics

▪ Comprehensive investigation of patients up to the point of intervention in the DGH setting

▪ Urgent increase in human resources in all disciplines required to achieve set standards for thrombolysis and revascularisation

▪ More highly specialised nurses in multiple settings.

There is a strong evidence base for the targets of the NSF, but the resources currently available in the UK are insufficient to achieve them, let alone the advances in practice demanded by evidence following the NSF in publication.[5,6]

WORK OF CONSULTANT CARDIOLOGISTS

1 Direct Patient Care

A Work in the specialty

The exact pattern of working will vary from area to area. The exact composition of services in a particular hospital, in terms of its referral patterns and the services it can provide vary so much that it is impossible to stipulate one particular pattern of care. The comments below are therefore generalised guidelines.

Inpatient work Regular ward rounds are essential with a consultant lead service. The frequency of the ward rounds will depend upon how sick the patients are. Patients admitted to hospital should be seen by a consultant within 24 hours. Consultants will normally carry out ward rounds at least twice a week and in addition will go to the wards on most days to see patients who are particularly unwell. In areas of high dependency, such as ITU and CCU, a daily consultant ward round (at least) is necessary.

Referral work   Referral work is carried out by consultants on a day-to-day basis as it occurs.

Inter-specialty and interdisciplinary liaison   Liaison is very important with other physicians involved in the care of the patient and in tertiary centres with the cardiac surgeons involved in the care. Furthermore there is a liaison with other specialised teams, depending upon the patient's illness, eg a patient with endocarditis would be seen by the cardiologist, the infectious diseases or microbiology team and there would also be involvement with the cardiac surgeons in case cardiac surgery was required.

Case conferences   Formal case conferences are not normally an issue in cardiology. They are occasionally required for particularly complex cases. Case discussions of difficult cases are frequent and carried out on a regular basis in order to answer clinical questions and also as a learning exercise.

Numbers of patients   The number of inpatients under the care of a consultant cardiologist will vary between hospitals and between secondary and tertiary care, with fewer, more complex, predominantly elective admissions in tertiary care and a greater number of emergency admissions in secondary care. No more than 20 inpatients should be under the care of a consultant cardiologist but this is often exceeded by demand.

Outpatient clinics   The pattern of outpatient work varies from hospital to hospital. In all, there are general cardiology outpatient clinics but in many hospitals there is a trend, at the present time, to set up rapid access clinics to deal with many of the patients who in the past attended a conventional type of clinic by appointment. These are particularly applicable to chest pain and are becoming ubiquitous. In other centres however there is rapid access to heart failure and arrhythmia clinics. There are also specialised clinics for patients with GUCH, lipid disorders, and in some centres, clinics for intractable angina.

The numbers of patients seen in conventional outpatient clinics would normally be 5 or 6 new patients or 12 to 15 review patients. The latter number may need review with the complexity of some follow-up patients.

Acute and non-acute general medical clinics   Most consultant cardiologists in secondary care take part in the acute medical take and will therefore be required to follow-up some of these patients in the outpatients department. Most patients will be discharged to the care of their general practitioner but some non-cardiac patients will be referred on to the appropriate medical specialty. (See also Acute Medicine, below.)

Specialised investigative and therapeutic procedural clinics   There are few such clinics in cardiology although in some areas pre-admission clinics for patients being admitted for cardiac catheterisation, pacemaker insertion and intervention are being established. These clinics are set up in such a way that there is plenty of time for the patient to have the procedure explained to them and to give their informed consent. Many of these clinics are nurse led.

The members of the multidisciplinary clinical team

The multidisciplinary team is central to the delivery of cardiac care. It comprises nurses, technicians and doctors, aided by clinical managers. The nurses' role is both on the ward and in outpatients. Nurses are becoming increasingly specialised and they may under supervision run chest pain clinics, heart failure clinics or be involved in the assessment of patients prior to investigations. Technicians carry out investigations involving electrocardiograms, exercise testing and echocardiography. Cardiologists oversee these investigations and are involved in the interpretation of them. Furthermore they carry out the clinical assessment of patients in both acute and chronic situations. They are responsible for carrying out procedures such as cardiac catheterisation and intervention and arranging for referral of patients on for cardiac surgery. See also iv.

Services outwith the base hospital: conjoined services

Clinics are often carried out in other small hospitals where there is no cardiologist eg, small community hospitals, and very occasionally outreach cardiology clinics are carried out in GP practices. Domiciliary work is rare in cardiology since complex cardiology is more effectively carried out in the hospital and it is best to facilitate immediate access to the hospital when this is appropriate.

Hospice work There is a possible role for this in heart failure.

On-call for specialist advice and emergencies Specialists must be on-call to give advice to junior staff and in addition to see patients immediately, irrespective of the time, who present particularly difficult clinical problems. Consultants also have to come into hospital, out of hours to carry out emergency procedures, including echocardiography, transoesophageal echocardiography, insertion of pacing wires and central lines and in tertiary centres to carry out complex procedures such as PTCA as an emergency. The latter may become routine in secondary centres as invasive services in secondary centres increase.

Specialised facilities and services within the specialty

Cardiology depends very strongly on investigations. Unlike many other specialties where investigations are mainly 'subcontracted' to other specialists, eg to radiologists, cardiologists tend to carry out their own investigations. There is increasing sub-specialisation however within cardiology, with cardiologists referring to other cardiologists when the problem is a specialised one. A good example of this is the referral of complex rhythm problems to electrophysiologists. The main specialist services provided by cardiology are listed overleaf.

Primary care

Services provided in primary care include:

hypertension clinics

risk assessment (including measurement and lipids)

recording ECGs in some practices

Secondary care

This would normally provide:

an ECG department

exercise stress testing

echocardiography & transoesophageal echocardiography and possible stress echocardiography

myocardial perfusion imaging and radionuclide angiography (often in association with the X-Ray department)

Holter recording to detect cardiac arrhythmias and BP monitoring

pacing, both temporary and permanent

tilt testing to diagnose causes of blackouts

coronary angiography to diagnose the cause of chest pain

Tertiary centres

Tertiary centres would provide all the facilities found in a secondary centre and in addition would provide:

angioplasty

electrophysiology (including ablation and insertion of intracardiac defibrillators)

specialised forms of pacing, including anti-tachycardia pacing

cardiac surgery

The specialised facilities required include adequate space and technical staff combined with the correct equipment to perform the above. In both the secondary and the tertiary centre pacing facilities are required as well as the equipment for complex pacing follow-up. This requires a significant amount of technician time.

B Acute medicine

Most consultant cardiologists have on-take responsibilities for the care of unselected acute medical admissions. There needs to be continual assessment of case workload of cardiologists so that the level of commitment to general medicine can be re-assessed commensurate with the need to increase cardiological uptake of acute coronary syndrome patients. The development of chest pain units within medical assessment units may help to define the appropriate cardiological share of the emergency take-in for the future.

C Academic medicine

The role of the cardiologist in academic medicine varies according to the setting. In the DGH the cardiologist must be involved in teaching the whole of the cardiology team and also involved in setting up local research and audit projects. In a teaching hospital some cardiologists will have a smaller clinical responsibility than the DGH cardiologist and are more likely to run multidisciplinary research teams investigating specific research topics.

2   Work to maintain and improve the quality of care

This work encompasses duties in clinical governance, professional self-regulation, continuing professional development, education and training of others. For many consultants, at various times in their careers, it may include research, serving in management, and providing advice. All require consultant participation. Such work is described fully in Part 1 of this document. Its scope is summarised in the Appendix to Part 2. Management and advisory work are identified specifically in the Appendix.

WORKFORCE REQUIREMENTS

The previous estimate was that one cardiologist was required per 80,000 population (3.1 per 250,000). Implementation of the National Service Framework for coronary heart disease requires 1 per 50,000 (5 per 250,000).

The most recent annual census of consultant physicians carried out in September 2000 showed 616 WTE consultant cardiologists in the UK (approximate population 59.7 million, ie over 1 per 99,000). The numbers for England, Wales, Northern Ireland and Scotland are given in chapter 7 of part 1 of this document.

Editors note: *In 1999 there was insufficient information available to allow a more precise estimate of the workforce requirements in this specialty. This recent estimate provides a firmer basis for workforce planning but this too will need to be reviewed in the light of developments in practice and service delivery.*

References

1.   Hall R *et al.* Fifth joint report on cardiothoracic services. *Heart* (Suppl) in preparation.

2.   Department of Heath. The National Service Framework for Coronary Heart Disease, DoH, 2000.

3.   Royal College of Physicians. Working for patients: Part 1 A blueprint for effective hospital practice; Part 2 Job plans for specialist physicians.

4.   Clinical effectiveness and evaluation unit of the Royal College of Physicians, London. *Myocardial infarction national audit project.* London: RCP (in press).

5.   National Institute for Clinical Excellence. *Glycoprotein IIb/IIIa inhibitors.* London, NICE, 2000.

6.   National Institutes for Clinical Excellence. *Automatic implantable cardiac defibrillators.* London, NICE, 2000.

Clinical genetics

i Introduction: a brief description of the specialty and clinical needs of patients

Clinical genetics is a medical specialty that receives referrals of all ages from all branches of medicine and surgery. Specific clinical activities are diagnosis of genetic disorders, risk estimation, genetic counselling, and support and management, especially in the light of genetic test results. The specialty also has an increasingly important role in areas such as education of other professionals and the public, in drawing up guidelines to good practice, providing expert advice, and in research and development.

The objectives of a clinical genetics service may be summarised as follows.[1]

▪ For those persons who are affected or who are referred, to make the genetic diagnoses, pedigree analyses and estimates of risk necessary in order that genetic counselling is well informed and to guide preventive and therapeutic actions.

▪ To support the identification and surveillance of *relatives* who are at risk for serious genetic disorders, but who may not have been directly referred in order that genetic counselling is well informed and to guide preventive and therapeutic actions, if required.

▪ To provide support to family members, both those affected and those who are not.

ii Organisation of the service, ways of working, clinical networks and community arrangements

Clinical geneticists work within regional genetic centres and, together with genetic counsellors and scientists, provide genetic services to the population of a defined geographical region. These services are delivered through a network of central, joint and district clinics. In each region there are strong links with genetic laboratories, oncology and fetal medicine centres, and with community and primary care teams. In most genetic centres about half of the referrals are from general practitioners and the remainder from other hospital specialties and other agencies.

The regional genetic centres have formed a national network to provide information and diagnosis for patients and families with extremely rare genetic disorders. Clinical genetic services are organised on a 'hub and spoke' model.[2] The regional genetic centre is the hub for the service and contains a range of core services. Locally based clinics and their support staff (secretarial and genetic co-workers) link closely with the regional centre.

Clinical genetics is mainly an outpatient specialty. When the consultant team receives a referral, a genetic co-worker (genetic counsellor) may contact the family before the clinic visit, to gain further information, including the family history, and to confirm medical details. Many referrals concern genetic disorders and complex malformation syndromes that call for precise diagnosis and calculation of risk. Other referrals are for common recessive disorders, trisomies, chromosomal translocations, and single gene congenital malformations. Often these are straightforward and genetic co-workers may take responsibility for assessing them. The training of such genetic counsellors is being developed nationally with a registration scheme in development.[3] A team approach to genetic referrals is the norm, which may need the skills of all the professionals in a regional genetic centre.

Genetic services have close links with other specialties, particularly cancer services. Some regions operate a system whereby patients complete a family questionnaire. Families identified as being at low risk of having a genetic cause for the particular cancer are seen by the local clinician for surveillance. High risk families are referred to the genetics clinic for assessment, and DNA predictive tests where these are available.

A number of centres undertake disease specific clinics and actively manage the surveillance for complications in specific disorders.

Most genetic centres (if not all) keep family-based records, using a dedicated computer system. They administer their own appointments system and request medical notes from other hospitals to confirm diagnoses. Summary letters are sent to patients and referring clinicians after clinic appointments. Administrative and secretarial staff are, therefore, integral members of the genetics team.

iii   Outline of clinical work of consultants in the specialty

Clinical geneticists are physicians who have undergone specialty training in genetics after general professional training in medicine or paediatrics (and sometimes in other specialties, such as psychiatry, obstetrics and gynaecology, ophthalmology). Specialty training covers a broad range of sub-specialties, such as the genetics of adult and paediatric disorders, cancer, dysmorphology, and neuropsychiatry. It also includes basic theoretical genetics, counselling theory and practice, laboratory experience and research. The Clinical Genetics Society has delineated the core responsibilities of a clinical geneticist.[4] They are as follows.

- Diagnosis of genetic disorders affecting all ages and body systems, birth defects and developmental disorders;
- investigation and genetic risk assessment;
- genetic counselling;
- predictive testing for late onset disorders using agreed protocols;
- where appropriate, follow-up and support and co-ordination of health surveillance for specific genetic conditions;
- where appropriate, the offer of genetic services to extended families;
- where appropriate and where sufficient resources exist, maintain genetic family register services;
- liaison with genetic laboratories;
- participation in national genetic networks;
- education and training of genetic professionals and other health care professionals;
- being a resource of expertise and information for the specialists, primary care doctors and other health professionals.
- research – clinical, biomedical, psychosocial and service related.

In this developing specialty the work of a clinical geneticist should be responsive to changes in service need.

iv Work of other members of the multidisciplinary team

Genetic co-workers

Genetic co-workers (genetic counsellors) are nurses or genetic associates with specialist training. In some units they hold their own clinics, with support and advice from consultants, for which consultant time should be allocated.

Laboratory genetic services

The clinical team works in close liaison with genetic laboratory staff, especially over the indications for and interpretation of extremely specialised genetic tests which may need to be tailored specifically to a particular family's clinical problem. Joint clinical and laboratory meetings discuss case management.

Other specialists

Many genetic units hold review meetings/clinics with other specialties such as radiology, fetal medicine, neurology, paediatric specialties.

v Facilities required

A clinical genetics service should be part of a regional genetic centre, with full access to specialised genetic testing laboratories and the University Department of medical genetics. The facilities required for clinical genetics services have been set out in a report from the Royal College of Physicians,[2] and are summarised below.

Facilities required to deliver a high quality clinical genetic service

Clinical facilities
Appropriate and sympathetic outpatient area suitable for families and for adult and paediatric patients;
Access to full range of outpatient investigations
Access to inpatient facilities for investigations (specific beds not required)

Office facilities
Adequate office space for consultant, other medical, co-worker and administrative/clerical staff
Secretarial support for clinic and other activities
Facilities for family record storage and retrieval
Library area for books, journals, database searching

Information and IT requirements
Computer facilities for genetic registers (dedicated)
Desktop computer facilities and links to allow searches of internet-based and other databases
Software for malformation and other diagnostic databases
Regularly used journals, books

General
Facilities for communicating between 'hub and spoke' parts of the service
Support for travel of medical/nursing staff for peripheral clinics, home visits
Adequate study leave for national meetings, inter-regional audit

vi   Quality Standards

Quality standards for clinical genetic services are discussed in documents from the Royal College of Physicians[1] and the British Society for Human Genetics.[5] Not all centres are able to operate in the same manner. This principally reflects historical differences in staffing levels, the geographical locations of the units and the distribution of the populations served. Most centres usually provide:

- pre-consultation assessment;
- clinical consultation;
- post consultation follow-up;
- in patient consultations;
- long term contact and review of high risk individuals by genetic registers;
- an urgent referral service for cases involving prenatal diagnosis.

The chief factor influencing access to service appears to be the availability of clinical genetics professionals.

WORK OF CONSULTANTS IN CLINICAL GENETICS

1   Direct patient care

A Work in the specialty

Outpatient clinics

New patient clinics   Depending on the complexity of the case and whether or not genetic co-workers have been involved beforehand, a consultation normally takes 45 minutes, and occasionally an hour. A consultant working alone is usually able to see three or four new families in a session of one NHD.

Specialist clinics   The number of patients seen depends on whether pedigree information is available beforehand, whether investigative procedures are carried out, and whether the consultant works alone or with other specialists. The arrangements should be agreed locally.

Follow-up clinics   Follow-up is often required to discuss the results of genetic tests and the implications. Each consultation might take 30 minutes. Without genetic co-workers more consultant clinics may be needed. In a new service most patients are first referrals, with few follow-up patients.

Review and recall   Many units have active review and recall systems, supported by genetic registers and dedicated staff. The purpose of this form of anticipatory care is to inform individuals and families of technical advances and new information for health interventions, reproductive decisions and life planning. Other units provide such a service within their routine working. Sessions for this work should be agreed locally.

Travel

District clinics allow equitable access to the service. Some are distant from the centre and there must be allowance for travelling time.

Junior medical staff

The work that can be undertaken by junior medical staff depends on their experience, and most new entrants have no experience in the specialty. A consultant must set aside time to supervise their work. Overall the contribution of a junior doctor might increase the amount of work that can be done in the clinic by 50%.

Supporting genetic co-workers

It is part of the work of consultant clinical geneticists to give support and advice to genetic co-workers.

Clinical discussion and laboratory liaison meetings

Attending regional and national clinical meetings (for instance to discuss rare cases of dysmorphic syndromes) is necessary to ensure quality of clinical opinion. Joint clinical and laboratory meetings to discuss case management are an integral part of a consultant's work and should be recognised as a (fixed) commitment.

On-call for occasional emergencies

Sessions must be allocated for emergency diagnostic work in early pregnancy. Some units also provide an emergency dysmorphology service to paediatricians.

Teaching, training and education

The work of a clinical geneticist includes a large commitment to education, involving professional and non-professional groups.[8] It may be appropriate for a consultant in the regional genetics centre to have dedicated sessions to co-ordinate and organise teaching and training activities.[10] Increasing the educational provision for other health service professionals has been identified as an urgent national need to enable adequate provision of services to families.[9]

Research

In a rapidly developing specialty where there are far more questions than answers, research forms an inherent part of the clinical geneticist's role. There is unanimity amongst practitioners that participation in research is essential to good clinical practice and that research activity should be broadly defined and not restricted to grant funded or laboratory projects.[4] Legitimate research activities include clinical delineation and study of natural history, biomedical, psychosocial, service delivery etc. and can all be performed either individually or in collaboration.

It is important that consultant contracts and work plans reflect and acknowledge research demands.

B Contribution to acute medicine

Clinical geneticists do not participate in the on-call rota for acute general medicine. They do, however, provide a consultation service for urgent problems (see above).

C Academic clinical geneticists

The NHS workload of academic clinical geneticists depends on their academic responsibilities and individual job descriptions. Most academic clinical geneticists make a strong contribution to the routine work of the NHS department in addition to providing tertiary services. Major advances in clinical research have come from the close collaboration between clinical geneticists, laboratory scientists and the patients who attend genetics clinics.

2   Work to maintain and improve the quality of care

This work encompasses duties in clinical governance, professional self-regulation, continuing professional development, education and training of others. For many consultants, at various times in their careers, it may include research, serving in management, and providing advice. All require consultant participation. Such work is described fully in Part 1 of this document. Its scope is summarised in the Appendix to Part 2. Management and advisory work are also identified specifically in the Appendix.

WORKFORCE REQUIREMENTS FOR CLINICAL GENETICS

Clinical genetic services involve medical staff and co-workers. Co-workers may be clinical nurse specialists or genetic associates with specific training in genetic counselling. The role and manpower requirements for such staff are set out in a College report.[6] This recommended a staffing level of two whole time equivalent (WTE) consultants and four co-workers per million populations as a minimum for a general genetic service. (This does not include a cancer genetics service). Figures from the South West of Britain Audit and Training Group based on actual referral rates per million population support this figure for a general genetic service. Service developments that are now generating a major additional workload – such as cancer genetics, and the need for the regional genetic services to undertake a large programme of genetic education – need additional manpower.

The requirement for a cancer genetics service has been identified as at least one consultant clinical cancer geneticist per million population.[11]

The most recent annual census of consultant physicians carried out by the College in September 1999,[7] showed 61 WTE consultant clinical geneticists. There is a need for planned expansion, co-ordinated with Specialist Registrar training posts. The number of trainees opting for part time consultant posts is increasing; figures in August 2001 presented to the Joint Committee on Medical Genetics suggest that 1.5 training posts are required for each WTE consultant post.

NOTE: *In 1999 there was insufficient information available to allow a more precise estimate of the workforce requirements in this specialty. This recent estimate provides a firmer basis for workforce planning but this too will need to be reviewed in the light of developments in practice and service delivery.*

References

1. Royal College of Physicians. *Clinical genetic services. Activity, outcome, effectivess and quality.* London: Royal College of Physicians, January 1998.

2. Royal College of Physicians. *Commissioning clinical genetic services.* London: Royal College of Physicians, December 1998.

3. Skirton H, Barnes C, Guilbert P, Kershaw A, Kerzin-Storrar L, Patch C, Curtis G, Walford-Moore J. Recommendations for education and training of genetic nurses and counsellors in the United Kingdom. *J Med Genet.* 1998;35(5):410–2. http://www.agnc.co.uk/training.htm

4. *The role of the clinical geneticist.* Clinical Genetics Society 2000: http://www.bshg.org.uk/Society/cgs/cgs.htm.

5. *Towards clinical governance in clinical genetic practice.* British Society for Human Genetics, 2000, Birmingham http://www.bshg.org.uk.

6. Royal College of Physicians. *Clinical genetics services into the 21st century.* London: Royal College of Physicians, 1996.

7. Royal College of Physicians. *Summary of information: consultant workforce in medical specialties in England ,Wales and Northern Ireland, 1999.* London: Royal College of Physicians, 2000.

8. Genetic Interest Group. Guidelines for genetic services. London: Genetic Interest Group, 1998.

9. Zimmern R, Cook C. The Nuffield Trust. *Genetics and health: policy issues for genetic science and their implications for health and health services.* London:The Stationery Office, 2000.

10. Report of a Working Party on Genetic Education to the Joint Committee on Medical Genetics. http://www.bshg.org.uk/jcmg/jcmg.htm

11. Department of Health. *Genetics and cancer services.* Report of a working group of the Chief Medical Officer. London: DoH, 1996.

Clinical neurophysiology

i **Introduction: a brief description of the specialty and clinical activity**

Clinical neurophysiologists undertake a variety of recordings and measurements of the electrical activity of the central and peripheral nervous systems. This information can be used to aid the diagnosis and management of a wide range of neurological conditions in all age groups. Activity is usually divided into four areas.

Electroencephalography (EEG)

The electrical activity of the brain (the EEG) can be recorded using either scalp (surface), or in special circumstances, intracranial electrodes. The majority of studies are undertaken on an outpatient basis using scalp electrodes. Recordings may last from a half to several hours, particularly if a period of sleep is included. The principal indication for EEG is in the investigation of epilepsy and other disorders of consciousness. Since it is rare for brief recordings to capture a clinical attack, these EEGs are usually referred to as inter-ictal recordings. Inter-ictal EEG is used to classify the type of epilepsy or seizure disorder and to provide evidence to support a diagnosis of epilepsy.

EEG activity now includes more specialist studies such as ambulatory EEG and video telemetry monitoring. These studies monitor EEG for several days in an attempt to capture a clinical attack and characterise the associated EEG. Some patients, particularly those being considered for surgical treatment of intractable epilepsy, may require intracranial electrodes (depth or sub-dural electrodes) as part of video telemetry EEG studies.

EEG are also used in the diagnosis and management of other conditions such as encephalitis, Creuztfelt Jacob disease, coma and neurodegenerative disorders including dementia. EEG studies may also be undertaken during neurosurgical procedures, to monitor cerebral activity, identify particular areas of cortical function and assist in the placement of deep brain stimulators in patients with intractable movement disorders.

Electromyography (EMG) and nerve conduction studies (NCS)

NCS recordings are made using electrical stimulation of the peripheral nerves. EMG activity measures the spontaneous and voluntary electrical activity produced in skeletal muscle. Many general medical disorders, as well as neurological disorders and trauma can cause damage to the peripheral nervous system. EMG and NCS identify and characterise the site and nature of the pathological processes affecting the peripheral nervous system.

Evoked potential studies (EP)

These studies are used to monitor the response of the peripheral or more commonly central nervous system to a variety of sensory or cognitive stimuli.

Intra-operative monitoring (IOM)

Monitoring evoked potentials, and in some cases EEG and EMG/NCS, can be used to protect various neurological structures and systems during neurosurgery or orthopaedic surgery. Monitoring can also be used during functional neurosurgery for disorders such as Parkinson's disease and pain relief surgery to identify the correct neural structures for stimulation and lesioning.

ii   Organisation of service

Clinical neurophysiology is largely a consultant provided service. The majority of neuro-physiological investigations are undertaken by consultant clinical neurophysiologists supported by trained neurophysiology technicians. In general, NCS/EMG and IOM procedures are undertaken by medical staff. EEG and EP examinations are performed by technical staff and the results reviewed and reported on by consultant clinical staff. Some senior technical staff also undertake NCS testing under consultant supervision. There are currently 31 SpR posts in the UK for the training of future consultant clinical neurophysiologists, but no junior staff at SHO level.

Most consultant clinical neurophysiologists are based in neuroscience centres or larger district general hospitals with neurological services. Many consultants also cover local district general hospitals from their bases in the tertiary referral centres on a hub and spoke model. A few consultants are based in larger district general hospitals with academic or teaching links to their local Neuroscience centre.

Neurophysiological testing requires provision of appropriate recording equipment and trained technical personnel. Therefore neurophysiological services are only usually available in tertiary referral centres or larger district general hospitals.

The majority of investigations are carried out on an outpatient basis. However, some patients with severe neurological or medical/surgical conditions may require treatment and investigation as inpatients, and studies may be undertaken in intensive care units or special care baby units.

iii   Special patterns of referral

Most patients are referred for investigation from other hospital consultants, principally neurologists, general physicians, rheumatologists, paediatricians and orthopaedic surgeons. Some neurophysiology departments provide access for general practitioner referrals but this is usually limited to specific conditions or indications.

iv   Requirements for a high quality service

Accommodation

The provision of an adequate neurophysiology service requires appropriate accommodation, testing equipment, technical and other support personnel.

The modern neurophysiology department should be a self contained unit with provision for patient reception, clinical investigation rooms and office space. Scattered rooms located on wards or corridors do not provide an adequate or safe environment for a quality neurophysiology service.

Clinical rooms should be of sufficient size to accommodate the testing equipment, examination chairs or couches, patients, medical and technical personnel together with the patient's carers and/or relatives. There must be suitable access for disabled patients or inpatients transferred on ambulance trolleys or beds. The department should also contain suitable, separate office space for consultant and technical staff and also accommodation for secretarial and administrative support staff. Neurophysiology departments should be sited for ease of access for outpatients who form the bulk of the patient workload. It is also important to site testing equipment well away from heavy electrical switch gear which might preclude satisfactory recording. Departments undertaking video telemetry monitoring should be within easy reach of the monitoring suite.

Medical staffing

The consultant clinical neurophysiologist should not work in isolation. The larger departments may contain two or more consultant neurophysiologists. Smaller DGH units, which may support only a single consultant, should have close links with a nearby larger clinical neurophysiology department. Each department should be led by a consultant clinical neurophysiologist supported by a senior member of the technical staff. The number of technical staff required will depend upon the workload of the department. For reasons of continuity of patient care and safety no department should be staffed with less than two (whole time equivalent) technicians. Larger departments will require three or more trained technical staff and should be large enough to support a programme of technician training.

Technical staffing

The provision of suitably trained and qualified technical staff is essential for the safe and efficient operation of a neurophysiology department. There is a national shortage of suitably trained technicians and the numbers of technicians entering basic grade training has fallen in the past five years. It is important that larger departments, especially those in regional neuroscience centres, develop basic grade training programmes and attract suitably qualified and motivated applicants to these training places. It is also important that larger departments also provide continuing post basic training, particularly in the more advanced areas such as video telemetry or intraoperative monitoring.

Administrative and secretarial staffing

Neurophysiology departments should also be equipped with adequate information technology to support an appointment and reporting system. This system should also provide a statistical information regarding activity and waiting lists. There should be adequate secretarial and administrative support for the consultant neurophysiologists and technical staff undertaking the various studies. There should be one WTE secretary per seven consultant clinical sessions. Departments should set standards for waiting times for investigation and processing times for report generation and dispatch. The Department should provide a system to prioritise requests, usually divided into urgent, soon or routine. Further subdivisions may be helpful, for example carpal tunnel screening clinics.

Equipment

It is essential that all departments have sufficient neurophysiology equipment to undertake the required EEG/EP or EMG activity. It is important that equipment is regularly tested for safety and accuracy. Many departments have now converted to digital EEG recording with significant advantages for storage, retrieval and transmission of data. This latter aspect is particularly important for smaller departments where there may not be a consultant neurophysiologist present on every working day.

v   Clinical work of consultants in neurophysiology

The working pattern of individual consultant neurophysiologists will depend upon their specialty interests and the local demands of the service. A few consultants, usually in specialist centres, may concentrate solely on either EEG or EMG/NCS investigations. Most neurophysiologists undertake a mixture of EEG/EP and EMG activity. This may include 3–4 clinical sessions for EMG/NCS studies in outpatients, and $1/_2$–1 sessions for inpatient EMG studies. A further 2–3 sessions will be required for EEG and Evoked Potential reporting. One session per week should be allocated to continuing medical education and audit. The pattern of on-call duties varies with local demands but urgent investigations are usually be uundertaken within 24 hours.

Some consultants with particular specialty interests, for example epilepsy, may participate in outpatient specialist neurology clinics, in collaboration with neurological colleagues. Consultant neurophysiologists who do not have dual accreditation with neurology or general (internal) medicine should not undertake general or specialist neurological clinics alone, or participate in acute medical take.

vi   Multidisciplinary team working

It is important that there are regular meetings and reviews between users of neurophysiological services and the medical and technical staff who carry out the neurophysiological studies. In centres undertaking complex surgical treatment for patients with epilepsy this may involve multidisciplinary meetings between neurologists, neurosurgeons, neuroradiologists, neuro-psychologists and neurophysiology staff. Similarly, departments undertaking EMG and nerve conduction study testing may require multidisciplinary meetings between neurologists, paediatricians, and muscle and nerve histopathologists. In smaller centres or district general hospitals which do not require multidisciplinary meetings, there should still be regular audit and review of activity between the referring clinicians and the neurophysiology department.

vii   Acute medicine

Neurophysiologists are rarely directly involved in the delivery of care in acute general internal medicine (see v above).

viii   Academic medicine

The NHS workload of academic neurophysiologists depends on their academic responsibilities and individual job descriptions, but in general academic neurophysiologists are an important component of a complex and technological discipline. Advances in the understanding of neurophysiological function of the nervous system are an important part of developing practice and academic appointments make a strong contribution to the work of the NHS departments.

In general most academic neurophysiologists will need at least 2–4 sessions devoted to academic work rather than NHS service activity. Academic appointments should not include any significant sessional commitment outside the regional or academic centre. It is important that academic departments have sufficient technical and support staff, possibly including engineers and information technology specialists to support clinical academic research.

ix Quality standards

Waiting time standards

To provide a quality service for patients it is important to set standards for waiting and reporting times. The following guidelines would provide an acceptable minimum standard of service for most departments:

■ For routine investigations, waiting times for EEG and evoked potential studies should be less than four weeks, and less than six weeks for EMG/NCS.

■ More urgent cases should be seen within two days for EEG and one week for EMG.

■ Urgent inpatient cases for both EEG and EMG should be seen within 24 hours.

WORK OF CONSULTANTS IN NEUROPHYSIOLOGY

1 Direct patient care

A Work in the specialty

Outpatient clinics

The number of outpatients seen per EMG/NCS clinic will depend upon the complexity of the investigations required. Usually, between four and six patient appointments would be expected per clinic session. This number should be reduced if the consultant is required to supervise concomitant carpal tunnel or peripheral nerve testing clinics undertaken by suitably trained technicians, or if supervising specialist registrars undertaking their own EMG/NCS clinics.

A consultant undertaking an EEG reporting session might be expected to report between 15 and 20 routine outpatient inter-ictal EEGs per session ($3^1/_2$ hours). This would include paediatric EEG studies and short-term sleep studies. The number of the EEGs reviewed per session should be adjusted downward if there is a significant teaching element for specialist registrars and technicians attending the reporting session.

The number of long-term ambulatory or video telemetry studies that could be reported in a session will depend on the degree of data analysis carried out by the recording technician. If there has been significant editing and data selection then four to six studies could be assessed per session. If the consultant does all data analysis, only one or two studies could be assessed per session. It is a good practice to involve the recording technicians in all consultant EEG reporting sessions.

B Acute medicine

Neurophysiologists are rarely directly involved in the delivery of care in general internal medicine (but see v above).

C Academic medicine

Most academic neurophysiologists need at least 2–4 sessions devoted to academic work. Academic appointments should not include any significant sessional commitment outside the regional or academic centre. It is important that academic departments have sufficient technical and support staff, possibly including engineers and information technology specialists to support clinical academic research.

2 Work to maintain and improve the quality of care

This work encompasses duties in clinical governance, professional self-regulation, continuing professional development, education and training of others. For many consultants, at various times in their careers, it may include research, serving in management, and providing advice. All require consultant participation. Such work is described fully in Part 1 of this document. Its scope is summarised in Appendix 1 of Part 2. Management and advisory work are identified specifically in the Appendix.

WORKFORCE REQUIREMENTS FOR NEUROPHYSIOLOGY

Consultant NHDs required to provide a service to a population of 250,000

Neurophysiology is predominantly an outpatient specialty and the following calculations are therefore based on the workload in the outpatient department.

Workload generated by a population of 250,000

The expected workload would be 800 EEGs, 600 EMGs, and 200 EPs per annum. From the activity figures quoted above this requires 40 EEG sessions, 120 EMG sessions and 10 EP sessions per annum – a total of 170 clinical sessions.

Other NHDs are required for:

- Special interest clinics, eg epilepsy, neuromuscular diseases – say 1 NHD and for:
- Administration, audit and management – say 1–2 NHD
- CME/CPD – say 1 NHD
- Teaching, training, clinical research – say 1 NHD (variable)
- Travel, depending on local arrangements – $\frac{1}{2}$–1 NHD.

Assuming that the consultant works alone, for 42 weeks per year (six weeks annual leave and four weeks study leave) this requires 317 (170 clinical + (42 × 3.5) non-clinical) sessions per annum. That equates to 1.1 (317/294) consultant neurophysiologists per 250,000 population (1/227,000).

The most recent figures from SWAG (July 2000) indicate that, in England and Wales, there were 71 whole time equivalent consultant neurophysiologists in post, with ten vacant posts. (It is also recognised that many potential consultant posts are not established or advertised because of a significant shortage of suitable applicants). There were 31 SpR (NTN) posts. It was estimated that to increase the total number of consultants to 108 by 2008 there would need to be two additional SpR posts each year from 2001–2003 inclusive; ie 6 posts. Currently no additional funding for these six posts has been approved. Current estimates are that there will be only 95 consultant neurophysiologist posts by 2008. Assuming a population of 46 million for England and Wales the total number of consultant neurophysiologists required to meet the above levels of activity would be 203. Given the current levels of funding and availability of training it is unlikely that this number will be achieved within the next 20 years.

Many neurophysiology departments have long waiting lists, particularly for EMG and Nerve Conduction Studies, and the demand for neurophysiological investigations is likely to increase. There is likely to be a significant adverse impact upon the quality of care for patients with acute or chronic neurological diseases or injuries to the nervous system. The serious gap between demand and supply will also lead to increasing numbers of tests being undertaken by unqualified or untrained personnel, with all the attendant risks to patient care and medico-legal claims which this will entail.

The calculations made above do not include the increasing demands for specialist iinvestigations, such as video telemetry for epilepsy surgery programmes, or intra-operative monitoring and detection. These developments will be severely limited by the lack of suitably qualified consultant neurophysiologists.

NOTE: *In 1999 there was insufficient information available to allow a more precise estimate of the workforce requirements in this specialty. This recent estimate provides a firmer basis for workforce planning but this too will need to be reviewed in the light of developments in practice and service delivery.*

WORK PROGRAMME

The following work programme summarises consultant activity for several different settings.

1. Direct patient care

Work in the specialty[1]	Workload	NHDs allocated
Inpatient EMG clinic	3–4 patients	0–1
Outpatient EMG clinics	4–5 patients	2–3
EEG/EP reporting sessions	15–25 studies	2–3
Specialised services (eg video telemetry)	2–5 studies	0–1
Work out with the base hospital	(EMG or EEG as above)	0–3
On-call for specialist advice and emergencies	Variable	0–2
Work in acute medicine		
On-take, and mandatory post-take rounds	N/A	
In academic medicine	Depending on post	0–4
2. Work to maintain and improve the quality of care		2–4

[1]Normally some of these sessions are fixed times each week.

Clinical pharmacology and therapeutics

i   Overview of the specialty

The work programme of a consultant in clinical pharmacology and therapeutics varies greatly, depending on the job setting. Consultants employed within the NHS will usually work as general physicians, and about half of their time will involve the supervision of acute medical admissions, responsibility for medical inpatients and running outpatient clinics. These individuals will normally have another clinical specialty interest (eg cardiovascular risk management, toxicology) and will take a close interest in prescribing issues. The National Poisons Information Service is run almost exclusively by NHS consultants in clinical pharmacology and therapeutics.

At the time of the last College census, approximately two-thirds of consultants in clinical pharmacology and therapeutics held academic appointments within universities. While having a service commitment, many of these individuals will have a strong research emphasis in their work which will contribute to knowledge about drug actions and their clinical usage. They will also play an important role in the planning and delivery of undergraduate teaching in therapeutics.

Since the mission of the specialty is to improve the care of patients by promoting safe and effective use of drugs and evaluating drug therapy, many consultants will make wider contributions to the NHS clinical service. At a local level this may involve work on Drug & Therapeutics Committees, drug formulary management, creating prescribing guidelines and providing assessments of new products. At a national level, many of the positions within key bodies such as the National Institute for Clinical Excellence, the Medicines Control Agency, the Committee on Safety of Medicines, the Joint Formulary Committee overseeing publication of the British National Formulary, the Medicines Commission and adverse drug reactions monitoring (pharmacovigilance) schemes are occupied by consultants in clinical pharmacology and therapeutics.

Other clinical pharmacologists at consultant level are employed by the pharmaceutical industry and are involved in the development of new drugs and early clinical trials in patients. Some also hold joint appointments with academic units or trusts, a trend that is likely to grow in the future.

ii   Specialty job plans

This specialty review and job plan attempts to reflect these very varied patterns of working. It also recognises that most NHS and academic consultants are accredited in both clinical pharmacology and therapeutics and general (internal) medicine as their second specialty. However, the skills of clinical pharmacology and therapeutics are generic and fully applicable to other medical specialties. There are a small number of consultants who also practice in geriatric medicine, paediatrics, oncology, respiratory medicine, and cardiology, and it is likely that the number of such consultants will increase in the future as more varied training schemes are established. The following sections describe:

- The areas of work and responsibilities (direct patient care and supporting activities) of a consultant in clinical pharmacology and therapeutics.

▯ An appropriate workload for an individual consultant.

▯ The facilities that are necessary to support consultants in meeting their job plan objectives.

▯ The workforce requirements for consultants in clinical pharmacology and therapeutics.

▯ A model work programme for a consultant based in (i) a University teaching hospital or (ii) an NHS district general hospital.

iii   Facilities required to meet the objectives of the job plan

The facilities required by consultants in clinical pharmacology and therapeutics include the following:

▯ Inpatient medical beds (approximately 15–20) to support acute medical services with appropriate levels of nursing support.

▯ Junior staff support, including the presence of a specialist registrar to support the admission of unselected acute general medical cases.

▯ Outpatient facilities with access to clinical laboratory services and space for teaching.

▯ Clinical laboratory facilities, which may include access to special investigations, sometimes necessitating collaboration with other specialists (for example, clinical biochemists).

▯ Research facilities, which may include protected beds for clinical research together with appropriately trained nursing staff, laboratory facilities with technical support, or computer hardware for data management.

▯ Secretarial support both for inpatient and outpatient activities, and other managerial responsibilities.

▯ Office space, including areas for filing and a computer.

▯ Library facilities.

▯ Teaching facilities for undergraduates and postgraduates, including data projection.

▯ Facilities to support the training of specialist registrars, including research facilities and computer and word-processing support.

▯ Pharmacy drug information service.

▯ Study leave and support for continuing medical education.

WORK OF CONSULTANTS IN CLINICAL PHARMACOLOGY

1   Direct patient care

Inpatient work

These sessions are devoted to supervising the management of general medical patients together with the specialist work of the individual consultant. This work normally requires two ward rounds per week, at fixed times. The number of inpatients for which the consultant team is responsible should not normally exceed 20. Part of this time will also be devoted to inpatient referrals for patients with pharmacological or toxicological problems. Consultants expect to work in an adequately staffed ward with the appropriate facilities and ancillary services to care for a typical case-mix of general medical patients. They should have the support of at least one junior doctor who has completed general professional training.

Outpatient work

Outpatient sessions are for seeing new patient referrals, including emergency referrals, and follow-up after discharge from A&E or a hospital ward. Consultants normally provide this service with the support of junior staff, who will require supervision. It is reasonable to expect that the assessment of a new patient will take about 30 minutes and follow-up patients about 15 minutes. Trainees require more time. They should not work in isolation and the consultant must allow time for their supervision. A typical clinic might include 4–6 new patients and 10–15 follow-up patients. These sessions should include time for dictating clinic letters and administrative matters relating to the outpatient service.

Some clinical pharmacologists also provide specialist clinics, for example in cardiovascular risk management or epilepsy. Patients are sometimes referred with specific therapeutic, toxicological, or other drug-related problems.

Acute medicine: on-take and post-take rounds

Consultants participate in the on-call rota for the supervision of receiving and triaging acute emergency admissions. These duties should be undertaken with the support of an appropriate number of junior doctors including a specialist registrar. Acute general medical admissions should, ideally, be admitted to a medical admissions unit with appropriate staffing levels and access to emergency investigations. The on-call rota should not normally be more onerous than 1:5.

Each period of acute admitting must include a post-take ward round with the junior staff who were involved in the admission process. In some services two ward rounds may be required in a 24-hour period (constituting a further NHD when this requires a substantial out-of-hours commitment). Consultants who are responsible for the review of poisoned patients have more regular post-take ward rounds.

Medicines management

While supervision and management of general medical patients is a major direct contribution to the NHS service, most consultants in clinical pharmacology and therapeutics take on other roles that contribute indirectly to achieving local NHS service objectives and standards. They include:

- *Drug and therapeutics committees:* overseeing the use of drugs in both hospital and primary care;
- *Drug formulary management:* maintenance of a local formulary, which may be jointly agreed with local general practitioners;
- *Prescribing guidelines:* editing and facilitating the production of local prescribing guidelines for common medical problems;
- *Health technology assessment* which might include reviews of new and established drugs, for clinical- and cost-effectiveness; and
- *Audit of local drug utilization.*

There should adequate provision for these service commitments within a job plan.

Drug information services

Some consultants may provide a drug information service, often with the support of a clinical pharmacist. This may include a therapeutic drug monitoring service, an important role in advising on the management and prevention of medication errors; and advice on drug overdoses and the management of drug adverse effects. Most consultants support the activities of the Drug and Therapeutics Committee. Some consultants have a specialist interest in forensic pharmacology and provide expert advice in coroner's, criminal and civil cases.

2 Work to maintain and improve the quality of health care (see also Tables i and ii below)

Approximately two-thirds of consultants in clinical pharmacology and therapeutics hold academic posts which accounts for the particularly diverse contributions that the specialty makes to the delivery of healthcare. Consultants in major teaching centres play a large role in the design and delivery of teaching in therapeutics to medical students. For new medical graduates prescribing drugs is a major activity, and one that is associated with significant clinical risk. For these reasons therapeutics remains an important theme within any medical curriculum and requires appropriate support from clinical teachers. Clinical pharmacologists are also involved in the delivery of postgraduate training in therapeutics to other health professionals within the NHS, including general practitioners, nurses and pharmacists.

Research is a fundamental part of the work of many clinical pharmacologists. This may involve clinical research in patients and healthy volunteers, but some individuals will lead teams of laboratory based researchers. These drug-related research activities make an important contribution to the local and national NHS R&D strategy, providing important long term benefits for patient care. The success of these activities will depend on the availability of suitable clinical and laboratory areas, recognition of the need for protected research sessions, and the support of appropriately trained clinical and technical staff. Their expertise in drug-related research means that clinical pharmacologists often have an important role on (or chair) local and multicentre research ethics committees.

For consultants in clinical pharmacology and therapeutics many of the management responsibilities will flow from their activities in medicines management, eg involvement in drug and therapeutics committees, drug formularies, clinical guidelines development, and health technology assessment. Drug utilisation and adverse reaction monitoring are particularly appropriate topics for clinical audit, and clinical pharmacologists should be expected to take a lead role. All of these activities make an important contribution to achieving local objectives in clinical effectiveness, clinical risk management, and clinical governance. Clinical pharmacologists are likely to play an important role in auditing and investigating local drug-related incidents.

The particular importance of these aspects of a clinical pharmacologists' work should be reflected in the preparation of the job plan.

WORKFORCE REQUIREMENTS FOR CLINICAL PHARMACOLOGY

In the 2000 consultant census there were 55 consultants in clinical pharmacology and therapeutics, equivalent to 1 per 800,000 of the population. The following calculation reflects the numbers of consultants required to provide a high quality national service, with particular emphasis on medicines management, toxicology, and academic activities such as teaching and research. This workforce will also contribute to the care of unselected acute general medical admissions. The calculation takes into account several important trends:

▌ year-on-year increases in acute general medical admissions;

▌ difficulties in providing general medical cover because of the increasing burden on physicians running a specialty service (eg gastroenterology, cardiology);

▌ decreases in junior doctors hours of work;

▌ the likely impact of working time directives;

▌ drugs accounting for an increasing proportion of NHS expenditure (currently 15% of the total) together with pressures to prescribe newer, more expensive medicines;

▌ requirement to contain costs by adoption of agreed formularies, and rigorous assessment of clinical- and cost-effectiveness of new drugs.

▌ a planned 40% expansion in medical student numbers and opening of new medical schools.

On this basis it is estimated that the workforce requirement for consultants in clinical pharmacology and therapeutics is approximately 200. This number of consultants equates to:

▌ one consultant per district general hospital serving a population of 250,000 (with an expected annual drug expenditure of £50M);

▌ one consultant per 180 medical students in training (of whom there are there are now 36,000);

▌ three consultants per medical school (assuming that two-thirds hold academic contracts).

This figure requires an expansion in consultant numbers of at least 10% per annum over the next decade. Following the successful joint initiative of the NHS Executive and the Association of the British Pharmaceutical Industry, the number of trainees in clinical pharmacology has increased in the past few years. The scheme acknowledges the shortage of trained individuals, and their importance to the future use of drugs in the NHS and 25 specialist registrars expect to complete training by 2004.

NOTE: *In 1999 there was insufficient information available to allow a more precise estimate of the workforce requirements in this specialty. This recent estimate provides a firmer basis for workforce planning but this too will need to be reviewed in the light of developments in practice and service delivery.*

WORK PROGRAMME

The following tables summarise the range of activities undertaken by consultant physicians in clinical pharmacology and therapeutics with responsibilities in general (internal) medicine, the recommended workload, and the allocation of sessions which are considered to be a period of 3.5 hours or one notional half day (NHD). The job plan is based on a commitment of 10 NHDs per week although the working pattern of most clinical pharmacologists will involve considerably more NHDs. Suggested work programmes have been provided for consultants working in (i) a university teaching hospital, and (ii) a district general hospital.

Academic clinical pharmacologists will normally hold a full-time university contract (the full-time salary being paid by the university) and an honorary (unpaid) contract with the NHS. The honorary contract should cover not more than six sessions, no more than three of which should be fixed. The award of these concurrent contracts recognizes the contribution that academic consultants make, both directly and indirectly (eg medicines management) to the NHS clinical service. This arrangement also recognizes that the activities carried out on behalf of the NHS have value for the performance of teaching and research. The number of fixed commitments should be agreed by the consultant and the medical director in consultation with the Dean and Head of Department. The academic contract will normally include responsibilities for research, administration, and undergraduate teaching.

In some cases it will be the university that makes a fixed sessional commitment to the NHS service, allowing for more flexible participation of the academic staff in clinical duties.

(i). Example of the work programme of consultant physicians in clinical pharmacology and general medicine, working in a university teaching hospital, as notional half days (NHDs) per week.

Direct patient care

Activity	Workload	Clinical staff	NHDs	Conjoined services
Acute admissions[1]	Depends on – number of admissions – rota – junior staff support	Appropriate to the clinical workload – SpR – SHO – HO	0.5–1	Appropriately staffed medical admissions unit Ready access to emergency investigations
On-take and mandatory post-take ward rounds[1]	As above	As above	0.5	As above

Inpatient work
  Regular ward rounds[1]
  Referral work
  Radiology meetings
  Case conferences
  Student teaching
	Two ward rounds per week	As above	1	Appropriately staffed general medical ward
				Paramedical support services
				Secretarial support must be available for team members

On-call for advice and emergencies, eg toxicological advice eg research trials	Highly variable but may be nearly continuous in some cases	Supervised SpR support may be available	0–1	Poisons Unit National Poisons Information Service

Outpatient clinics
  General medical clinic[1]
  Specialty clinic[1]
	One G(I)M clinic per week
	  4–6 new patients
	  10–15 follow-up patients
	One specialty clinic
	  4–6 new patients
	  10–15 follow-up patients
		SpR support
		
		SpR support
			0.5–1	Radiology
				ECG
				Laboratory services
				Phlebotomy (hard pressed services)

continued over ▶

Direct patient care *(continued)*

Medicines management
    Drug & Therapeutics
        Committee
    Formulary
        management
    Prescribing
        guidelines
    Health technology
        assessment
	Overseeing the use of drugs in both hospital and primary care
	Maintenance of a local formulary which may be jointly agreed with local general practitioners
	Editing and facilitating the production of local prescribing guidelines for common medical problems
	Providing assessments of new and established drugs with analysis of clinical- and cost-effectiveness
		0–1	Administrative support
			Pharmacy information
			Clinical audit team

Specialised services eg drug information	Variable	0–1	Pharmacy

[1]Normally these sessions are at fixed times each week

Work to maintain and improve the quality of care

Activity	NHDs

Teaching and Training
    Undergraduate teaching
    Postgraduate training
	1–2

Research
    Clinical research
    Basic research
	1–4

Continuing Professional Development
    Continuing professional development
    Clinical audit
	0.5

Clinical Governance (Professional Self-Regulation)
    Lead clinician
    Team member
    Professional advisory groups
	0.5

Administration	1–2
Management and Advice	1

[1]Normally these sessions are at fixed times each week

Note: The total number of sessions worked by a consultant can be very variable. Most work programmes indicate an excess of 10 units worked. There will be times in the career of a consultant when management and national duties will be carried out to increase the number or sessions. Consultants who hold academic posts are likely to share clinical responsibilities with an academic colleague, halving the sessional commitment to the clinical service.

continued

(ii). Example of the work programme of consultant physicians in Clinical Pharmacology and General (Internal) Medicine, working in a general hospital, as notional half days (NHDs) per week.

Direct patient care

Activity	Workload	Clinical staff	NHDs	Conjoined services
Acute admissions[1]	Depends on – number of admissions – rota – junior staff support	Appropriate to the clinical workload – SpR – SHO – HO	1–2	Appropriately staffed medical admissions unit Ready access to emergency investigations
On-take and mandatory post-take ward rounds[1]	As above	As above	1	As above
Inpatient work Regular ward rounds[1] Referral work Radiology meetings Case conferences	Two ward rounds per week	As above	2	Appropriately staffed general medical ward Paramedical support services Secretarial support must be available for team members
On-call for advice and emergencies eg toxicological advice eg research trials	Highly variable but may be nearly continuous in some cases	Supervised SpR support may be available	0–1	Poisons Unit National Poisons Information Service

Outpatient clinics
General medical clinic[1]
Specialty clinic[1]
	One G(I)M clinic per week
	  4–6 new patients
	  10–15 follow-up patients
	One specialty clinic
	  4–6 new patients
	  10–15 follow-up patients
		SpR support
		
		SpR support
			1–2	Radiology
				ECG
				Laboratory services
				Phlebotomy (hard pressed services)

Medicines Management Drug & therapeutics committee Formulary management Prescribing guidelines Health technology assessment	Overseeing the use of drugs in both hospital and primary care Maintenance of a local formulary which may be jointly agreed with local general practitioners Editing and facilitating the production of local prescribing guidelines for common medical problems Providing assessments of new and established drugs with analysis of clinical- and cost-effectiveness		0–2	Administrative support Pharmacy information Clinical audit team
Specialised services eg drug information	Variable		0–1	Pharmacy

[1]Normally these sessions are at fixed times each week

continued over

Work to maintain and improve the quality of care

Activity	NHDs

Teaching and Training
  Undergraduate teaching
  Postgraduate training
	1

Research
  Clinical research
  Basic research
	1

Continuing Professional Development
  Continuing professional development
  Clinical audit
	0.5

Clinical Governance (Professional Self-Regulation)
  Lead clinician
  Team member
  Professional advisory groups
	0.5

Administration	1
Management and Advice	1

Note: The number of sessions worked by a consultant can be very variable. Most work programmes indicate an excess of 10 units worked. There will be times in the career of a consultant when management and national duties will be carried out to increase the number or sessions.

References

Royal College of Physicians. *Clinical Pharmacology and therapeutics in a changing world.* Report of a working party. London: Royal College of Physicians, 1999.

Royal College of Physicians. *Governance in acute general medicine. Recommendations from the Committee on General (Internal) Medicine of the Royal College of Physicians.* London: Royal College of Physicians, 2000.

Federation of Royal Colleges of Physicians of the UK. *Acute medicine: the physician's role. Proposals for the future. A working party report of the Federation of Medical Royal Colleges.* London: Royal College of Physicians, 2000.

Dermatology

i Introduction: a brief description of the specialty and clinical needs of patients

Dermatologists manage skin diseases in people of all ages. Most dermatologists are skin surgeons as well as physicians. Skin diseases are disfiguring, distressing and highly symptomatic. Chronic inflammatory skin diseases significantly reduce quality of life and they impose a considerable burden within the community.[1,2,3] About one in four of the population are affected by skin disease that would benefit from medical care. In the UK skin diseases are among the commonest certified causes of incapacity to work.

Between 1981 and 1991 consultations for skin disease in general practice rose by almost 50%. This reflected an increase in prevalence of common problems such as atopic eczema, venous leg ulcers and skin cancer as well as the availability of effective treatments.[3] GPs refer 1–2% of the population to dermatologists each year as new patients.

Teaching and postgraduate education are essential parts of the work of dermatologists, who teach and train medical students, postgraduates, GPs and nurses. Although about 15% of GP consultations relate to problems with the skin, only 20% of GP vocational training schemes contain a dermatological component; and the undergraduate curricula contains on average only six days of dermatology. Newly appointed GPs therefore have little experience of dermatological problems.

ii Organisation

Primary care and community dermatology

The delivery of dermatology services in England is being reviewed within a government programme, *Action on Dermatology*. It is likely that more care will come to be provided in the community, with liaison dermatology nurses, 'intermediate care' clinics and leg ulcer clinics.

Some GPs with expertise in dermatology provide an intermediary service for colleagues in primary care. The British Association of Dermatologists recommends that such services should be limited to specific procedures and to specific areas of management; for example, the management of venous ulcers or the treatment of patients with chronic inflammatory skin diseases. Such services should be developed in collaboration with local dermatologists, integrated with local services in secondary care and provided in adequately equipped and staffed facilities.[4]

Secondary care

Dermatologists provide a hospital-based service in departments with facilities for outpatients, skin surgery, day-care and inpatients. Consultants with appropriate support work chiefly in outpatient clinics or outpatient operating theatres. They also provide on-call cover for urgent problems and support for other specialists.

Dermatologists should not practise single-handed and hospitals serving a population of 250,000 need at least three consultant dermatologists with appropriate support staff, including specialist

▌ *An appropriate number of patient appointments at each clinic.* Recommendations are based on published studies.[6] A maximum of 12 patients per doctor (with trainees or students), or 15–18 patients (with no trainees) in a single consultant session.

▌ *Experienced dermatology nurses to assist in the clinic*

▌ *Dressings, topical treatments etc.*

▌ *A pharmacy service able to meet needs identified in the clinic*

▌ *Dermatology secretarial staff.* Secretarial staff should be adequately trained in dermatological terms and policies and provided with appropriate word-processing and data collection facilities to allow proper clinical audit.

▌ *Medical photography service.*

4. Day treatment unit

   Daytime, after-hours and weekend access to these services should be provided. The service should have:

   ▌ Specified area where topical treatments can be applied

   ▌ Suitable bathing and showering facilities

   ▌ Appropriately trained nursing staff.

   All PUVA units should be supervised by a named consultant, thus ensuring accuracy of dosimetry, record keeping and the training and monitoring of the staff who administer treatment. UV output of units should be monitored by a medical physicist.

5. Dermatological surgery

   A quality service should include:

   ▌ A specified dermatology operating theatre equipped with appropriate instruments and facilities

   ▌ Trained nursing staff

   ▌ A defined case load.

   There should be an agreed definition of a day case and recognition of the time required to perform the various surgical procedures.

6. Inpatient care

   ▌ Dedicated inpatient beds

   ▌ A quality contract should include the provision of dedicated beds, staffed by experienced dermatology nurses

   ▌ Each patient must be allocated a named nurse on admission.

7. Laboratory support services

   Dermatology requires the same support services as many other general medical specialties - for example, chemical pathology, haematology, X-ray; but it particularly requires services in immunology, immunopathology and histopathology.

8. Support of other hospital specialties

    Dermatology patients require access to other hospital specialties, including histopathology with specific expertise in dermatopathology, plastic surgery, radiotherapy, immunology, and psychiatry.

9. Patient support groups

    Patient groups are an important source of support for people with specific skin diseases. Their literature should be available and departments should display addresses and points of contact.

10. Discharge letters and future management plans

    When a patient is discharged from either inpatient or outpatient care the general practitioner should be informed of the patient's status, with advice on further management.

vi   Outline of clinical work in the speciality

Most consultant dermatologists spend between five and seven clinical sessions each week in outpatient departments (including a surgical session) or on the wards. They also supervise the care of patients attending for day-care treatment. Most consultants undertake regular ward rounds, including review of ward referrals. Those with expertise in subspecialties such as photobiology, paediatric dermatology, dermatopathology, or contact allergy testing may have one or more sessions for this work.

Surgery is an increasingly important part of the workload because of the rise in incidence in skin cancer and the two-week waiting list imperative for cancers. A limited number of surgical procedures, such as cryosurgery, curettage, simple excisions and biopsies may be done in the outpatient clinic, but larger surgical procedures are done in a dedicated theatre session. Many larger departments have appointed a dermatologist to take on complex cancer surgery, such as Mohs' surgery and laser surgery, and these dermatological surgeons may devote most of their sessions to cutaneous surgery.

Dermatologists supervise the care of inpatients including:

▓ those with severe skin diseases that require intensive management. Many have concomitant disease, and may be elderly or socially deprived.

▓ children on paediatric wards under the care of dermatologists and/or paediatricians.

▓ those with life-threatening problems; eg severe drug reactions, who may require admission to an intensive care unit or burns unit.

Some consultants spend considerable time travelling from one hospital to another, and may be expected to provide on-call service for ward referrals and emergencies in a number of different hospitals. Other consultants based in one hospital with colleagues and good support staff have a less onerous on-call commitment. The need for domiciliary visits varies in different communities.

vii Work of other members of the multidisciplinary team

Dermatology nurses

Nurses with expertise in dermatology are key members of the team.

- They counsel and treat patients in day-care units and on the wards, and provide phototherapy (PUVA and UVB), carry out contact allergy testing (patch-testing), and care for wounds and chronic leg ulcers.
- Specialist nurses working in outpatient departments may provide information to patients, demonstrate and apply treatments (in children as well as adults), dress wounds, remove sutures or review follow-ups.
- Nurses with training in skin surgery assist in operating theatres and provide advice to patients undergoing surgery. In some units appropriately trained nurses perform skin biopsies or other surgical procedures such as cryosurgery.
- Dermatology nurses may advise professional colleagues caring for patients with skin problems in the hospital and the community.
- Dermatology nurses, also trained in paediatrics, provide outreach services for children with problems such as atopic eczema.
- Liaison nurses who work in the dermatology department and in the community can help to provide a seamless service as well as assisting with the training of practice nurses.
- Liaison nurses may advise on the management of leg ulcers or attend community leg ulcer clinics.

Cosmetic camouflage

Trained Red Cross volunteers provide this service for patients with disfiguring skin lesions.

viii Conjoined services

These include:

- Dermatopathology and immunopathology
- Medical photography, medical physics, vascular technology
- Chiropodists, psychologists, tissue viability nurses
- Community leg ulcer clinics, patient support groups

ix Specialised facilities

Integrated facilities should be the goal for all departments. The physical proximity of inpatient, outpatient, and day-care facilities helps efficient working.

Outpatient unit

Outpatient units should provide:

- Dedicated outpatient area with rooms large enough for patient, consultant and medical students or other trainees
- Natural lighting and additional lighting

▪ Examination couches

▪ Wound dressing area

▪ Treatment rooms

▪ Facilities for contact allergy testing

▪ Refrigerator for storing contact allergens

▪ Rooms for patient education and educational material

▪ Medical photography services

▪ Pharmacy for preparation of topical medicaments and allergens for contact allergy testing

▪ Accommodation within the paediatric department for paediatric dermatology clinics.

Day-care centres and phototherapy

Day-care complements inpatient care. Day care centres should be in a position to provide an out-of-hours service, including phototherapy. Specialist dermatology nurses, who can provide skin care, rather than physiotherapists, should run phototherapy units.

▪ Phototherapy area with TLO1 and PUVA

▪ Treatment room; eg facilities for bathing or showering.

Surgical facilities

▪ Well lit operating rooms with couches

▪ Equipment for electrocautery, diathermy and hyfrecation.

▪ Equipment for cryosurgery and storage for liquid nitrogen

▪ Facilities for freezing biopsies and storing frozen samples

▪ Laser-safe areas where required.

Inpatient unit

All dermatologists should have admitting rights to a dedicated inpatient dermatology unit staffed by trained specialist nurses. Medical cover is provided by consultants and/or SHOs and specialist registrars. Patients with widespread chronic inflammatory skin diseases benefit from admission and are aided by the mutual patient support provided on a dermatological unit. Dedicated inpatient beds, some with facilities for reverse barrier nursing, are also required for patients with severe and life-threatening skin conditions. Teaching hospitals need dedicated inpatient dermatology units for tertiary referrals of patients with complex diseases; and also for the training needs of undergraduates and specialist registrars.

Two dedicated dermatological beds per 100,000 population are the minimum requirement, but eight beds are the minimum required to support appropriate staffing for a self-contained unit. The hub and spoke arrangement referred to in (iv) is often the most appropriate way of ensuring that dermatologists have access to a suitable dedicated dermatology inpatient facility. Dermatological beds in general medical wards are only satisfactory if there are appropriate facilities for bathing and treatment and patients receive care from specialist dermatology nurses.

Inpatient facilities

In a dermatological inpatient unit there should be:

▯ Dedicated dermatology beds

▯ One bed in a side room, with provision for isolation and photoprotection

▯ Adjacent bathing and showering facilities

▯ A treatment area.

x   Quality standards (see also Sections v, vi above)

The concept of a quality driven service, with standards of care clearly defined in contracts, provides a framework in which the quality of dermatology care for a community can be improved.[5] Standards should be set in relation to:

▯ the referral system

▯ outpatient clinics

▯ dermatological surgery

▯ outpatient / daypatient treatment

▯ inpatient care

▯ discharge from the dermatology service

▯ the training of medical and nursing staff

▯ the availability of appropriate facilities and equipment

▯ administration

▯ information for, and education of, patients

▯ storage and handling of medical records.

Contracts should incorporate protocols for referral and for shared care, treatment guidelines, and standards for audit and quality control. Other outcome assessments that might be used are quality of life and patient satisfaction.

xi   Contribution to acute medicine

Dermatologists provide a consultation service for urgent problems. Some patients, eg those with cellulitis or drug eruptions, may be admitted directly to the dermatology unit from the acute medical take. Dermatologists do not participate in the on-call rota for general medicine.

xii   Academic dermatologists

The NHS work of academic dermatologists depends on their academic responsibilities and individual job descriptions, but most academic dermatologists make a strong contribution to the routine work of the NHS department in addition to setting up tertiary services. Major advances in clinical research have come from the close collaboration of dermatologists, laboratory scientists and patients.

xiii Developments that offer improved patient care

- *'2-week wait clinics'* Patients with suspected skin cancer must be seen within 2 weeks of referral. This requirement may delay appointments for other patients with acute problems. The impact of the 2-week wait must be evaluated.

- *Dermatological surgery* This subspecialty has developed rapidly in response to the need to treat skin cancer efficiently and cost-effectively in outpatient clinics. Examples are 'One stop' tumour clinics with facilities for immediate skin surgery and the availability of Mohs' surgery for complex tumours.

- *Nurse-led outpatient clinics* These are an effective way of monitoring therapy and providing treatment.

- *Multidisciplinary clinics* These have improved the service for patients with complex problems.

- *Liaison nursing* Liason nursing by trained dermatology nurses has improved management of adults and children with inflammatory skin diseases by integrating primary and secondary care and has raised the standard of community dermatology.

- *Community leg ulcer clinics* With appropriate resources (trained nurses, dressings, compression bandages) have raised the standard of care in the community.

WORK OF CONSULTANTS IN DERMATOLOGY

1 Direct patient care

A Work in the specialty

Inpatient work

- *Ward rounds* with specialist nurses and other members of healthcare team: two per week Teaching and training are an important component of ward rounds.

- *Referral work.* Requests for a dermatological opinion are common. Ward referrals are seen on the wards or in outpatient clinics as required.

Outpatient work

The greater part of the work of consultant dermatologists takes place in outpatient clinics, the activities of which are set out overleaf.

General dermatology clinics:

Patient ratio: On average, 1 new to 2 follow-up patients

Average number: *i. No trainees*

> 15–18 patients per consultant per clinic. There is inadequate time when there are new patients with chronic diseases e.g. psoriasis, atopic eczema; complicated reviews (most reviews will be complex because simple problems should have been discharged to GP); skin surgery.

Average number: *ii. With trainees, students, non-training grades*

> 12 patients per doctor per teaching / training clinic
>
> Consultants train doctors (GPs, SHOs, specialist registrars) and nurses in outpatient clinics in both DGHs and teaching hospitals. One consultant can supervise a maximum of two trainees or non-training grades per clinic but must allocate extra time to review the patients and teach trainees and students.

Special clinics within dermatology:

- Tumour clinics ideally with facilities for immediate skin surgery (one-stop clinic)
- Vulva clinics with facilities for colposcopy
- Paediatric dermatology clinics in suitable paediatric facilities with paediatric-trained nurses
- Other multidisciplinary clinics depending on the expertise of the consultant dermatologist and the resources in the hospital (see iv above).

Specialised investigative and therapeutic procedure clinics:

- Dermatological surgery clinic including Mohs' micrographic surgery with dedicated surgical facilities suitable for day surgery (trained histopathology technician required for Mohs' micrographic surgery).
- Laser-surgery clinic. A laser-safe area is required and a general anaesthetic operating list for treatment of children with port-wine stains.
- Contact allergy and occupational skin disease clinics involving work place visits as well as allergy testing in the hospital department.
- Photobiology clinics with facilities for phototesting and "hotel" facilities for patients.
- Wound care (leg ulcer) clinic.

All clinics will require adequate support staff including specialist nurses. The number of patients seen depends on the complexity of the procedure or investigation.

Services outwith the base hospital (see Sections ii, iv above)

On-call for specialist advice:

Dermatologists provide a service for emergencies referred from the community and from other specialities.

B Acute medicine

Dermatologists do not participate in the on-take rota for unselected medical emergencies.

C Academic medicine

The NHS workload of academic dermatologists depends on their academic responsibilities and individual job descriptions, but in general academic dermatologists make a strong contribution to the work of the NHS department.

2   Work to maintain and improve the quality of care

This work encompasses duties in clinical governance, professional self-regulation, continuing professional development, education and training of others. For many consultants, at various times in their careers, it may include research, serving in management, and providing advice. All require consultant participation. Such work is described fully in Part 1 of this document. Its scope is summarised in the Appendix to Part 2. Management and advisory work are identified specifically in the Appendix.

WORKFORCE REQUIREMENTS FOR DERMATOLOGY

Dermatology is predominantly an outpatient specialty and the following calculations are based on the workload in the outpatient department.

For a population of 100,000

If 1.5% of a population of 100,000 is referred per annum this generates 1,500 new patients. With a ratio of 1 new to 2 follow-up patients per general clinic, 1,500 new patients plus 3,000 selected follow-up patients gives 4,500 patients per year.

Assume consultant works 42 weeks per year (6 weeks annual leave, 4 weeks study leave/professional leave and bank holidays).

Consultant working alone

4,500 patients per 42 weeks = 107 patients per week, which with 15 patients per clinic requires 7 NHDs. In addition at least two NHDs are required for one theatre list per week and a ward round per week. Other NHDs are required as follows:

Direct patient care:*	NHD
Weekly review of dermatopathology	$\frac{1}{2}$
On-call	$\frac{1}{2}$
Travel (variable depending on number of centres visited)	$\frac{1}{2}$–1
Work to maintain and improve the quality of care:	**2–4**
Administration, audit and management	1
CME/CPD	1
Teaching, training, clinical research (variable)	1

*This does not include consultants' special interests and the need for day-care, phototherapy, or patch testing, all of which are parts of a dermatology service.

Therefore the total sessional requirement for consultant dermatologists to serve a population of 100,000 is at least 13.0 NHDs.

For a population of 250,000

The requirement for a district general hospital serving a population of 250,000 to provide a clinical service in dermatology is 33 NHDs, ie one consultant per 85,000 population.

Consultant working with an assistant or trainee

The figures given above assume consultants are working alone. If in every clinic a specialist registrar or a general practitioner assisted under supervision, they could see 24 patients altogether in each clinic. The calculation applied above suggests a requirement for one consultant per 100,000 plus one whole time equivalent assistant. For a population of 250,000 $2\frac{1}{2}$ whole-time equivalent consultants plus $2\frac{1}{2}$ whole-time equivalent assistants are required.

Notes

1. *Ratio of one new patient to two follow-up patients*   It is difficult to discharge more patients if GP referrals are appropriate and the needs of trainees are considered. Knowledgeable GPs only refer complex problems that need specialist management. It is not possible to discharge these patients after one or two visits. Trainees must follow their patients to learn how to manage disease. Therefore when trainees are present, although the overall number of patients per clinic increases this has little impact on the number of new patients seen because the consultant will see fewer patients and trainees bring back more follow-ups. The ratio may approach 1:2.5 if phototherapy and patch testing are included.

2. *15–18 patients per clinic*   New patients who have difficult forms of common problems such as psoriasis or atopic eczema deserve more than a 10-minute consultation. Consultants certainly need more than 10 minutes when treating chronic diseases with potentially toxic therapy. It is possible to see more patients in a tumour clinic but only if surgery is not performed during the clinic.

3. *Each consultant works with one trainee and/or non-training grades*   No consultant should work in isolation from colleagues. All consultants responsible for a population of 100,000 should have assistance in clinics.

4. *Specialist services*   The pattern of work will depend on the specialist services provided by individual consultants and departments, eg skin surgery, contact allergy (patch) testing, wound healing, paediatric dermatology, phototherapy, dermatopathology.

Conclusion

It is clear why the British Association of Dermatologists recommends the equivalent of one whole-time consultant dermatologists per 85–100,000 population to cope with the need for specialist advice, ie an increase from 368 to 635 whole-time equivalent consultants in dermatology for England and Wales. But in autumn 2000, 65% of trainees are women. A target of 825 dermatologists by 2009 would allow for flexible patterns of working.

The specialty must expand at more than the historic 5% per annum to reduce waiting lists (which are 18 months in some Trusts), cope with the needs of patients with common problems such as skin cancer, and respond to increasing requests for training from medical undergraduates, postgraduate trainees, GPs and nurses. The England and Wales population of 52,000,000 needs at least another 300 consultant dermatologists.

Note: These calculations do not take into account the requirement that patients with suspected skin cancer be seen within two weeks of referral.

NOTE: *In 1999 there was insufficient information available to allow a more precise estimate of the workforce requirements in this specialty. This recent estimate provides a firmer basis for workforce planning but this too will need to be reviewed in the light of developments in practice and service delivery.*

References

1.   Williams HC. *Dermatology: Health care needs assessment* (Eds A.Stevens, J.Raftery). Radcliffe Medical Press, 1997.

2.   Harlow D, Poyner T, Finlay AY, Dykes PJ. Impaired quality of life of adults with skin disease in primary care. *Br J Dermatol* 2000;**143**(5):979–82.

3.   Williams HC. Increasing demand for dermatological services: how much is needed? *J R Coll Physicians Lond* 1997;**31**:261–2.

4.   Provision of secondary care for dermatology within general practice. *J R Coll Physicians Lond* 1999;**33**:246–8.

5.   Quality in the dermatological contract. A report from the Workshop on quality issues in dermatological contracting of the British Association of Dermatologists. *J R Coll Physicians Lond.* 1995;**29**(1):25–30.

6.   Savin JA. Validation of the recommendations on clinic size made by the British Association of Dermatologists. *Br J of Dermatol* 1997;**136**:968–971.

Diabetes and endocrinology

i   The specialty and the clinical need

Diabetologists and endocrinologists provide advice to people of all ages after childhood on a variety of metabolic and endocrine conditions. Type 2 diabetes is a progressive condition of adulthood which eventually develops in 10% of the UK population, and through its impact on arterial disease consumes some 8–10% of health care resources. Type 1 diabetes and other forms are much less common, but often difficult for the person with the condition to manage, lifelong. They may have devastating impact on visual, cardiovascular, renal and nervous systems if expert professional advice is not available.

Endocrine conditions are diverse in their requirement for specialist medical advice, but their impact is also lifelong. Many pose a diagnostic challenge, and in some the application of new but only partially effective treatments requires fine judgement. Endocrine disorders affect many body systems, and call for expertise in metabolic disease, clinical biochemistry, cardiovascular disease, neurology, disorders of the ear nose and throat, and others.

Endocrinology

Primary health care teams usually restrict their non-integrated input to endocrinological conditions into the continued management of hypothyroidism. However they will usually have an integrated role in the management of some of the complications of endocrinological conditions, such as hypertension, pain control, and psychological disturbance. Many endocrine conditions are uncommon and diverse in presentation, and diagnostic procedures are often arcane, complex (and changing). Inevitably, therefore, referral is sometimes delayed.

A major challenge to the endocrinologist is diagnostic planning. This often uses the latest of a variety of imaging techniques (requiring liaison with radiology and medical physics), ordering and interpreting hormonal investigations and provocation tests (which requires understanding of complex biochemical pathways, and the physiology of feedback systems). Endocrinologists must also have expertise in a smaller number of procedures (such as thyroid needle biopsy). Diagnosis is not always categorical, the conditions are lifelong, and many treatments are complex. This calls for skills in communication and counselling.

Endocrinological treatments are often non-curative and only partly effective, and sometimes there is none. They range from hormonal treatment to surgery and to radiotherapy, and may have diverse side effects. Choice of therapies, or even whether to advise treatment requires fine judgement and counselling, as does the planning and interpretation of the monitoring of therapy outcomes. Biotechnology increasingly offers new approaches to diagnosis and therapy. These include better genetic understandings of the basis of the autoimmune and oncological susceptibilities to endocrine disease, and new opportunities for family counselling.

Type 1 and secondary diabetes

Insulin therapy remains a complex and difficult area of clinical pharmacology, and indeed is becoming more so with the advent of new insulins with new pharmacodynamic properties. There is increasing recognition of the need to reach glucose control targets to prevent the devastating late complications of the condition. Very few primary health care teams find they have the expertise to manage this condition.

Referrals are nearly always pre-diagnosed, and indeed have often been managed for some years by paediatric diabetologist. Adult physicians and the diabetes team should work closely with their paediatric equivalents. Diagnostic skills are only rarely required. The principal clinical management skill is in adapting the inappropriate pharmacokinetics of a wide range of insulin preparations, with different effects in different individuals, to a diverse range of variable lifestyles. As an optimal outcome is rarely achieved and the results adversely affect aspects of daily living, skills in communication and counselling are at a premium. A good outcome requires closely integrated activity with other members of the diabetes team, notably diabetes specialist nurses and dieticians. Team management skills are also at a premium. The failure of insulin therapy means that structured care organisation to detect complications as they develop is also mandatory, necessitating good organizational management skills.

Type 2 diabetes

Many primary health care teams are organised to manage patients with the condition. However, many patients also require specialist advice at critical moments in the disease process. Therefore the disease is increasingly managed as the paradigm of integrated care, with common protocols and support systems. Unfortunately, at present the strains on primary health care are resulting in increasing numbers of referrals for routine care to secondary care centres.

Type 2 diabetes is primarily a metabolic condition, with principal impact on the arterial wall. The main skills in management are firstly in counselling and behavioural modification, to enable the person affected to improve their lifestyle skills; and secondly in the optimal management of blood lipid, blood pressure and blood glucose control. This calls for skills in preventive cardiovascular medicine and an understanding of knowledge-based medicine and its application.

Only limited diagnostic skills are required, but optimum prevention of late complications requires skills in the organisation and conduct of surveillance. Because of the integration of care with primary health care, the specialist in this area often needs extensive health care management skills; for example, to deliver retinal screening services to a population and district-wide quality development and monitoring systems. This implies close working with colleagues and managers in primary health care, and participation in the work of groups charged with organising care.

As with Type 1 diabetes, care is multidisciplinary (with podiatry an important element).

Other metabolic services

Diabetes specialists are expert in cardiovascular prevention, and often provide local specialist lipid services alongside clinical biochemists. Some diabetes specialists work with specialists in other metabolic disease in adults; for example, in the management of cystic fibrosis, and in obesity services.

Acute general medicine

The general aspects are covered elsewhere. Specialists in diabetes and endocrinology expect to deal with some hyperglycaemic emergencies (both new diagnoses of diabetes and known diagnoses), the occasional intractable hypoglycaemic problem, and more uncommonly an Addisonian crisis or thyroid crisis/coma.

Associations for people with endocrinological conditions

Diabetes has a long history (>60 years) of consumer led activities. Local groups often appreciate a continuing input, and often leadership, from their local specialist.

ii Organisation of care

Endocrine services

Most of the clinical activity is in secondary care and is outpatient based. Dedicated day or overnight investigational facilities are needed to support this, usually employing designated nursing staff working to endocrinological protocols. Inpatient beds are required for difficult investigational problems, conditions complicated by other disease, and for courses of therapy requiring special administration techniques or needing special monitoring.

There must be access to sophisticated imaging techniques, and to hormonal and biochemical investigations, although these are usually available in any NHS sub-region. Patients with rare or complex disorders, such as infertility or endocrinological malignancy, are often referred to colleagues with a supra-specialist interest. Outpatient services are usually divided into supra-specialties, particularly where joint clinics are held with other specialties such as thyroid oncology, eye clinics and reproductive services.

Advances in provision of support services mean that most hospitals can provide an endocrine service, but often there is referral to sub-regional centres.

iii Ways of working

Diabetes services (see also Box 1)

As noted above, diabetes services are increasingly provided as an integrated district-wide service, but the involvement of primary health care practices is diverse. People referred to secondary care are generally seen in a secondary care diabetes centre by a dedicated multidisciplinary team. Where primary health care services are well developed (and the identified load of people with management problems therefore high), the numbers of referrals and people needing advice can be high (about 5000 per 250,000 population). To be effective, clinical management must be structured, and almost entirely outpatient-based. It requires team protocols, standardised record forms, recall support for annual review surveillance, education provided by nurse specialists, careful triage of patients whose feet are damaged or at risk with timely referral to podiatry, and dietetic education and advice.

The diabetes centre with its multidisciplinary team is the major specialist facility. Within the centre a clinical database collecting annual review data as a minimum is an essential requirement for quality development purposes. Increasingly, and with due mechanisms to protect confidentiality, this extends to provide the district diabetes quality development system. The diabetes centre will also provide, and organise recall for, the district diabetes eye surveillance system, static or mobile or both.

Inpatient care for people with diabetes is mainly concerned with ensuring safe and optimal practice to those admitted unwell or for procedures to other specialist services. Because of the high prevalence of diabetes after middle age (6–10%), this can be a large workload. Few specialist diabetes beds are required, though patients need specialist care for an ischaemic or infected foot or the infrequent hyperglycaemic and hypoglycaemic emergencies.

Obstetric services for women with diabetes are usually provided jointly in obstetric outpatient clinics with a dedicated obstetrician. The diabetes physician may be the focus for advice on other general medical problems in pregnancy. Support is also be required for maternity units.

iv   Components of care provision

Outpatient services

New referrals in endocrinology   These are to confirm or exclude a wide range of endocrinological conditions. They generally require a complete history and examination, and ordering of investigations specific to the condition suspected. An investigation plan for tests as a day case may be devised, or arrangements made for tissue biopsy. In some cases the suspect diagnosis can be excluded on the basis of history/examination, but follow-up with review of findings is needed. There must be sufficient time for explanation and discussion with the patient. A new referral takes about 30 minutes.

Follow-up services in endocrinology   These are for review and discussion of previous findings, planning any further investigation, or planning or review of treatment (efficacy and problems). Again there must be sufficient time for explanation and discussion of progress and prognosis. A follow-up appointment takes about 15 minutes.

Special clinics in endocrinology   These may include thyroid eye and thyroid cancer clinics, pituitary clinics, and reproductive services. Often a second specialty is involved in such services, and discussion with the other consultant is a part of the service. Care provision and the time needed are as for other endocrine clinics.

New patient clinics in diabetes   These are for confirmation of diagnosis followed by a review of the lifestyle factors (Type 2 diabetes) contributing to the condition, or the lifestyle factors (Type 1 diabetes) which will have an impact on self-management with insulin. A general history and examination excludes other contributory illnesses. A specific history and investigations determines arterial risk level. Examination/retinal photography confirms the presence or absence of late complications. The person with diabetes then is taken to see the specialist nurse/dietician for further education and advice on self-management skills. Allow 30 minutes of consultant time.

Follow-up clinics in diabetes   These are for multiproblem consultations. They deal with lifestyle achievements and problems pertaining to blood glucose, body weight, blood lipid, renal function and blood pressure control (± smoking); review of progress to individual targets in each area, review of therapies in each of these areas; review of complications from the therapies (especially hypoglycaemia), and review of management of complications (especially foot care). Appreciation of the *multicultural factors* affecting health care is important. Allow 20 minutes consultant time.

Box 1: A framework of diabetes care

Ensure provision of the following:

A diabetes team (professionals) with up-to-date skills, including:

- doctors
- diabetes nurse specialists/assistants and educators
- nutritionists (dieticians)
- podiatrists (chiropodists)

A solid infrastructure

- easy access for people with diabetes
- protocols for diabetes care
- facilities for education and foot care
- information for people with diabetes
- structured records
- recall system for Annual Review/eye surveillance
- access to quality-assured laboratory facilities
- database/software for quality monitoring and development
- continuing education for professional staff

A range of services

- for regular review (often 3-monthly)
- for Annual Review
- for education
- for foot care
- for eye surveillance
- emergency advice line
- access to heart, renal, eye, vascular specialists
- joint obstetric service

A system for quality development

- feedback from people with diabetes on service performance
- regular review of service performance

From: International Diabetes Federation. A desktop guide to type 2 diabetes mellitus. *Diabetic Med* 1999;**16**:716–30.

Annual review clinics in diabetes   For multidisciplinary consultation, including eye, foot, and renal assessments, review of cardiovascular disease and events, symptoms of complications of diabetes, blood pressure, injection sites, diabetes knowledge and skills, pregnancy risk, and possible confounding conditions. The consultant's role is usually to assess the findings of the team, adding to them in the medical area, and developing and discussing the management plan for the next 12 months. Allow 15 minutes of consultant time.

Joint obstetric clinics in diabetes   Provide the special and intensive care needed by pregnant women with diabetes, ideally when conception is being planned. Held in conjunction with nurse specialists from both disciplines, and obstetricians. Weekly clinic with a variable load.

Special and other joint clinics in diabetes   In some services dedicated clinics are provided, with or without the presence of other specialists, for the management of conditions such as foot problems/vascular disease, diabetic renal disease, or young people's diabetes. Provision depends on the pattern of local care arrangements.

Inpatient services

Specialist advice Endocrinological and diabetes requests for review of inpatients vary according to the size of hospital served and provision of specialist services (eg ENT, neurology, obstetrics) within it. Peri-surgical management protocols can reduce the need for specialist diabetologist involvement, while improving care. Similarly, diabetes specialist nurses and dieticians can often deliver the care needed by the newly diagnosed inpatient, who can then be formally assessed in the new referral outpatient clinic. Patients using insulin will make effective use of a telephone service, which is usually team based.

Specialty admissions Endocrine patients admitted for sophisticated or complicated investigations generally require consultant review of their management, with planning of further investigations or therapy. This often involves discussion with colleagues in radiology, surgery and other specialties. An investigation unit with a high level of activity will also require its own weekly ward round and case review. Diabetic foot problems require daily to twice weekly consultant review, and often discussion with vascular surgical colleagues. Diabetes emergencies are usually managed within the context of acute medical services.

v Quality development

Quality development is well developed in diabetes services. It is based on national datasets that have been aggregated into clinical databases. These can be analysed to determine how well process and outcomes of care meet recommended target levels. It is an Audit Commission expectation that this work is done within services and incorporated into national diabetes care assessment packages. A consultant diabetologist is normally expected to lead on this activity. This work might take 0.5 NHDs consultant time per week.

Local work to improve the quality of care

This is addressed as a generic issue elsewhere in this document, and includes local management and CPD activities common to all specialties.

District diabetes management

Additionally to generic management requirements community leadership is required from any diabetes service. Many districts have appointed a community diabetes specialist, or at least someone with sessions dedicated to that role. The activities will include:

▮ chairing or being the major resource for the local diabetes planning group (LDSAG or HImp)

▮ devising and agreeing protocols of care common to primary and secondary care

▮ providing limited outreach clinics to assist in the establishment of primary care based services

▮ providing medical supervision to community diabetes specialist nurses

▮ ensuring the provision and development of dietetic and podiatry services in the community

▌ supervising the development of a shared district diabetes IT system and its use in quality development

▌ supervising support services provided by the diabetes centre for the community, such as retinal recall and surveillance mechanisms.

vi   Activities beyond the local services

The modern NHS has a large appetite for national and regional expertise in all specialities, not least in diabetes and endocrinology. These currently include:

▌ supervision of postgraduate training (regional-SpR programmes)

▌ structure of postgraduate training (SACs)

▌ inspection of postgraduate training

▌ development of clinical governance tools

▌ development of quality monitoring tools

▌ *NICE* guideline development

▌ driving (etc) and diabetes advice

▌ *NICE* technology appraisals

▌ provision of CPD programmes.

vii   Acute medicine

Both diabetes and endocrinology are chiefly outpatient specialties with a small inpatient load. These consultants are not ward-based, and a high acute medical load is inefficient and quickly leads to excessive hours of work. Nevertheless endocrine diseases and diabetes may particularly affect the cardiovascular and neurological systems and it is desirable that consultants in the specialty take part in any acute medical rota that is not fully supported by acute medical specialists.

With ward rounds, post-take rounds, an allowance for time on call, and follow-up activity, a 1 in 21 rota can be accommodated in 1.5 notional half days (NHDs) per week. Increased NHDs are required if on-call time is more frequent.

viii   Academic activities

Education and training activities are discussed elsewhere in this document. Consultants working in hospitals allied to university medical schools are usually expected to have additional responsibilities for university related activities and research, irrespective of the actual employer. The extent of this activity varies between consultants. It may encompass administrative responsibilities locally or nationally, as well as research programmes and non-clinical teaching. Academic physicians engaged in research will normally be expected to spend a limited amount of time in the dissemination of the results of that research outside their own locality.

Both diabetes and endocrinology are active foci of basic and clinical research, and there have been dramatic effects on health care delivery in the last 20 years. Diabetes is also a major focus of health care development internationally, with similar gains.

WORKFORCE REQUIREMENTS FOR DIABETES AND ENDOCRINOLOGY

Specialist medical workload

The tables that follow refer to responsible doctor (consultant) time requirement in the secondary care sector. They do not attempt to quantify total medical or other clinical contacts for people with diabetic or endocrine conditions.

Most patients referred to secondary care will require other attendance to be reviewed by non-consultant members of the team as required. This is in contrast to practice in other Western European countries where nearly all follow-up contacts will be by registered specialists.

Background

Calculated time requirements reflect increasing patient numbers (diagnosed prevalence) and changes in practice. Improvements in care have become necessary especially in the light of the better medical and economic evidence that adverse health outcomes of high cost are preventable, and that such activity is cost-effective.

Account need to be taken of the extra quality development (audit) and district diabetes management activity of diabetes consultants, although this latter will vary considerably between individuals. Account also needs be taken of the typical consultant time requirement for CPD, training of specialist registrars, senior house officers, and house physicians, and in training/education of other members of the health care team including GPs. Many specialists are also involved in clinical research.

Relevant *changes in pattern* of diabetes practice include:

▮ Diabetes is becoming more common as the population ages, with about 10% of 70-year-olds affected; typical prevalence is now 2.4% (assuming small ethnic minority community).

▮ There is increased case ascertainment with heightened primary care awareness of diabetes.

▮ There is better case ascertainment of complications through provision of structured services in primary and secondary care.

▮ Increased evidence that tight control reduces complication rates in both Type 1 and Type 2 diabetes has lead to increased referral to consultants for intensification of metabolic control.

▮ There are effective methods of managing high-risk feet and early diabetic nephropathy.

▮ Diabetologists are increasingly involved in care of patients with lipid disorders; an area driven by new evidence of effective care.

▮ Integrated locality diabetes care requires leadership, training, and team management beyond those found in other medical specialities, these usually falling to the local specialists as the only people with the relevant expertise.

▮ Increasingly, much endocrinology is being referred to local hospitals rather than teaching centres, with an increase in the workload of physicians previously primarily appointed as diabetologists.

Calculations:

Diabetes activity

Assumptions:

1. Based on a non-teaching district with active integrated diabetes care and a high level of primary health care involvement.

2. The evidence base is that with highly development primary health care, around 40% of people with diabetes require secondary care management. There is a tendency for this to increase in the last year or so, due to pressure on primary health care services, but this has not been factored in.

3. Support from a well-developed diabetes care team, with adequate provision of diabetes specialist nurses, podiatrists, dieticians, and retinal screeners. Not yet the case in most of the UK, but moving that way.

4. Out-of-clinic activity is taken as being 50% of the total in-clinic time. Based on local experience.

5. Consultants with typical annual leave, study leave, plus small contributions for illness and official leave.

6. Every patient in secondary care sees the responsible consultant once per year as a minimum, and 25% more often. However, the majority of consultations are with other team members.

7. Joint obstetric services, but no formal joint clinics otherwise.

8. Diabetes service management centred on one individual consultant, but with input from others into management of parts of the service (eg retinal screening) and divided liaison with GP-based services.

Table 1. Predicted new and review attendances in diabetes per 250,000 population.

	Year	
	2000	**2005**
Number of patients (n (% prevalence))	6,000 (2.4)	6,500 (2.6)
Review patients		
Number requiring hospital review (x 1/yr)	2,400	2,600
Number requiring >1 visit per year	600	650
Time requirement (hr at 15 min/patient)	750	812
New referrals	1,400	1,516
Time requirement (hr at 30 min/patient)	700	758
Time requirement (out-of-clinic patient activity, hr)	725	785
Total time requirement (hr/yr)	*2,175*	*2,355*
Total time requirement (hr/wk, 42 week year)	*51.8*	*56.1*

Table 2. Time requirement (hours/week) for predicted diabetes specialist clinic activity, diabetes service management, ward work, and inpatient consultations per 250,000 population.

	Year	
	2000 (hr/wk)	**2005 (hr/wk)**
Specialist clinics		
Foot / pregnancy / renal / adolescent	14.0	15.2
Resulting out-of-clinic activity	7.0	7.6
Inpatient activity – regular	14.0	15.2
Hospital inpatient consultations / surgical	14.0	15.2
Management of local diabetes services	7.0	7.6
GP liaison	3.0	3.2
Total time requirement (hr/wk)	*59.0*	*63.9*
Deflator for 42 week year	*73.0*	*79.1*

Endocrinology activity

Assumptions:

1. Based on a non-teaching district with modern imaging and clinical biochemistry services.

2. Activity is many times higher in teaching centres – when calculating total need for endocrinologists a multiplier of 5 for 20 centres (ie a 50% increase in time requirements country-wide) is probably appropriate.

Table 3. Predicted new and review attendances in endocrinology per 250,000 population.

	Year	
	2000	**2005**
Review patients		
Number having secondary care attendance	1,550	1,700
Time requirement (hr at 15 min/patient)	387.5	425
New referrals	280	325
Time requirement (hr at 30 min/patient)	140	162.5
Time for out-of-clinic activity (hr)	263.8	293.7
Total time requirement (hr/year)	791.2	881.2
Total time requirement (hr/wk, 42 week year)	18.8	21.0
Day care investigation/procedures/consults (hr/wk)	4.8	4.5
Total time requirement (hr/wk)	*23.6*	*25.5*

Synthesis: **Diabetes and endocrinology clinical activity**

Table 4. Summation of pure diabetes and endocrinology clinical activities as hours per week per 250,000 population (from Tables 1, 2 and 3).

	Year	
	2000 (hr/wk)	**2005 (hr/wk)**
Diabetes mainstream outpatient	51.8	56.1
Diabetes other	73.0	79.1
Endocrinology	23.6	25.5
Total	*148.4*	*160.7*

Work to maintain and improve the quality of care:

In full, 8.5 hr/wk which, with a 42 week year, is 10 hr/wk. This should be allocated to acute general medicine on a proportional basis. At 50% of time this would be 5 hr/wk.

Total supra-specialist requirements:

On the basis set out above, the total requirement per 250,000 population is 153.4 hours per week, or 4.0 consultants working 38.5 hours per week. This figure will rise to 4.3 consultants by 2005.

Total consultant requirements including acute general medicine:

This depends on the acute general medical input of these individuals. While the multiplier is often 3.0 in non-teaching districts, with adequate staffing of other supra-specialties it might fall to 1.5.

WORK OF CONSULTANTS IN DIABETES AND ENDOCRINOLOGY

It is obvious that individual workloads vary enormously with the mix of diabetes, endocrinology and acute general medicine, and local and national management activities. However an average work distribution can be calculated for illustrative purposes, as shown below.

▪ Acute medical work at low intensity during working hours (see section vii)	1.5 NHDs
▪ Rota allowance for acute medical activity at low intensity, plus on-call commitment, both with SpR	2.0 NHDs
▪ Clinical governance, self-regulation, education and training, research, management and advice (elsewhere in this document)	3.0 NHDs
▪ Diabetes and endocrinology activities (10–6.5)	3.5 NHDs
Within this 3.5 NHDs the average distribution of activity will be:	

diabetes mainstream outpatients	42%
diabetes special	33%
endocrinology	21%

Gastroenterology

i   Introduction

The specialty of gastroenterology and hepatology cares for patients with disorders of the gastrointestinal tract and the liver. The specialty encompasses a wide range of conditions from frequent common disorders to highly specialised complex problems such as transplantation.

Common problems include indigestion, reflux, the irritable bowel and constipation. Much of the work is outpatient based, to exclude organic disease in the symptomatic patient. Investigations often include endoscopy and imaging. An acute inpatient service is needed for common problems such as gastrointestinal haemorrhage, jaundice and abdominal pain. More specialised units are required for the treatment of gastrointestinal cancer at all sites, the management of peptic ulcer and reflux, small bowel disease, inflammatory bowel disease, disorders of the hepatobiliary tree and liver. A small number of units undertake organ transplantation, including transplantation of the liver and small intestine.

ii   Organisation of the service

Most symptomatic patients are looked after by their family practitioner, and between them most problems are resolved by discussion, advice and medical treatment. Most other problems can be resolved by appropriate outpatient medical or surgical referral. Some patients require emergency inpatient care, particularly those with abdominal pain, gastrointestinal haemorrhage or acute colitis, and a smaller number require admission for evaluation of persistent symptoms.

While much of the inpatient work is broad-based there is increasing specialisation within gastroenterology. There is co-location of medical and surgical working for treatment of disorders of the oesophagus and stomach, hepatobiliary and pancreatic disease, disorders of the liver, small bowel disease and of medical/surgical groups concerned with the treatment of colorectal disease. Each of these groups plays a major role in the investigation, diagnosis and treatment of cancer at each of these specific sites.

iii   Special patterns of referral

Outpatient referral is now more targeted. For example, there are clinics for patients with specific symptoms as dysphagia, jaundice, rectal bleeding or abdominal pain. Primary care referral to hospital based open access endoscopy is also a common pattern of referral.

iv   Ways of working

Close links have been created with primary care particularly to ensure appropriate patient referral. Community arrangements are essential for patients discharged on supplementary enteral or parenteral nutrition.

v   Requirements for a high quality service

While most of the patient care takes place in the outpatient department, with outpatient investigation, this must be supported by a combined medical and surgical inpatient unit for acute and elective problems within gastroenterology, particularly acute abdominal pain, gastrointestinal haemorrhage and acute colitis. Specialist units have been developed at both district and teaching hospital level, with some regional and national centres for specific problems.

The main service groupings are for upper gastrointestinal disorders, including the oesophagus and stomach, hepatobiliary and pancreatic units, and colorectal units. Regional and national units include those for acute and chronic liver failure and transplantation, particularly of the liver and small intestine.

The key features of a high quality service in the specialised units are co-location of the medical and surgical practice, with a team approach of the specialists, dietitians, nutrition specialists, and close collaboration with colleagues in imaging and histopathology and laboratory services.

vi   The work of consultants in the specialty

The clinical commitments are providing inpatient and outpatient services in general medicine, gastroenterology and hepatology, a specialist diagnostic and therapeutic endoscopy service, and facilities for nutritional support. Gastroenterology is characterised by high volume, frequent outpatient consultations, and several sessions per week in diagnostic and therapeutic endoscopy, together with the inpatient care of patients within acute medicine and the specialty. There are regular collaborative meetings to discuss clinical problems. Other tasks include contributions to the teaching and appraisal of medical staff and teaching medical students, continuing medical education, clinical audit, clinical research, administration and management.

vii   Multidisciplinary working

The workload is shared with a wide variety of colleagues in nursing, dietetics, nutrition, imaging and histopathology. This team effort is a hallmark of the specialty.

viii   Conjoined services

The chief complementary services include, nurse specialists, stoma therapists, nutrition nurse specialists, and dietitians.

ix   Specialised facilities

The specialised facilities include a diagnostic and therapeutic endoscopy unit, facilities for parentral nutrition, and in complex units, such as liver transplantation, a wide range of facilities including operative, anaesthetic and intensive therapy unit support. There must be arrangements to support close collaboration with colleagues in oncology.

x   Quality standards

Quality standards in most areas of gastroenterology have been developed by the British Society of Gastroenterology. Up-to-date guidelines for all branches of the specialty are available from the Administrative Secretary, British Society of Gastroenterology, 3 St Andrews Place, London NW1 4LB. The National Institute for Clinical Excellence (NICE), 19 Longacre, Covent Garden, London WC2E 9RZ, website www.nice.org.uk has issued guidance on a wide variety of gastrointestinal topics (including, for example, the use of proton pump inhibitors and treatment of dyspepsia, and guidance on the use of Ribervirin and Interferon alfa for hepatitis C.

xi   Developments that offer improved patient care

There are many opportunities for improved patient care including clear guidelines for the management and primary care of patients with peptic ulcer and non-ulcer dyspepsia. The increasing use of targeted outpatient clinics, the development of groups for patients with suspected malignancy, and joint medical and surgical assessment and management in all areas of the specialty. Other developments include major advances in diagnostic and particularly therapeutic endoscopy and major developments in imaging, particularly of the use of MRI and endoscopic ultrasound. Some invasive diagnostic procedures such as endoscopic retrograde cannulation of the pancreas are being replaced by MRI techniques. All these developments need to be underpinned by first class teaching and training and academic units working in close collaboration with those delivering the clinical service to ensure that the basic science and so that pathogenesis are adequately supported, encouraged and funded.

The identification of *Helicobacter pylori* as the cause of peptic ulcer and the cure of peptic ulcer with treatment for one week by triple anti-microbial therapy has been a remarkable example of such development.

WORK OF CONSULTANTS IN GASTROENTEROLOGY

1   Direct patient care

A Work in the specialty

The following describes the work of a consultant physician providing a service in acute general medicine and gastroenterology and recommends a workload consistent with high standards of patient care. It also sets out the work generated in gastroenterology by a population of 250,000, and gives the consultant workload as notional half days (NHDs) for each element of such a service.

The Royal College of Physicians Gastroenterology Committee and the British Society of Gastroenterology have published several studies concerned with the provision of a combined general medical and gastroenterology service. The most recent summarised the nature and standards of gastrointestinal and liver services in the UK.

The following account will apply to most consultant physicians in gastroenterology, although the pattern may be different in specialist centres.

The following guidelines and recommendations on the appropriate workload for each element of the consultant's work have been drawn up following extensive consultation within the specialty.

Inpatient services

A consultant-led team should look after no more than 20–25 inpatients at any time. Most are admitted on emergency 'take' days, with various general medical problems. A minority are admitted, either urgently or electively, for evaluation of gastrointestinal problems. NHDs need to be allocated for two routine ward rounds and one post-take ward round per week per consultant.

Outpatient services

New patient clinic A consultant physician in gastroenterology working alone in a new patient clinic sees 6–8 new patients in a session of one NHD, the number depending on experience and the complexity of the problem. Endoscopic procedures should normally be carried out at a different time, except for flexible sigmoidoscopy, which might in appropriate cases be performed at the same visit.

Outpatient review of selected patients following acute medical admission A consultant physician working alone in a follow-up clinic sees 15–20 patients in a session of one NHD.

Follow-up specialist clinic for chronic gastrointestinal and liver disease A physician sees 15–20 patients in a session of one NHD.

Junior medical staff support Outpatient clinics are often run with doctors in training, either SHOs or specialist registrars, and the consultant must allocate time to review the patients seen by them. The number of patients that junior staff see depends on their experience. For each junior doctor, the outpatient workload is increased by about 50% of that undertaken by the consultant. It should be noted that this only creates a potential saving in outpatient and endoscopy consultant sessions and not in the other components of the consultant's work. Moreover this saving (amounting to perhaps one session) is counterbalanced by the need for the consultant to devote time to training (including training in endoscopy).

Diagnostic and therapeutic endoscopy service The workload of a consultant physician undertaking endoscopy depends on the procedure, as follows.

Diagnostic upper gastrointestinal endoscopy/diagnostic flexible sigmoidoscopy A maximum of 10–15 procedures should be carried out in a session of one NHD.

Therapeutic upper gastrointestinal endoscopy endoscopy This includes injection sclerotherapy and banding of oesophageal varices, injection of bleeding ulcers, palliative treatment of oesophageal cancer, and placing feeding tubes (percutaneous endoscopic gastrostomy – PEG). Such procedures take twice as long as routine upper GI endoscopy and 5–8 might be undertaken in a session.

Therapeutic flexible sigmoidoscopy This usually involves polypectomy and takes twice as long as routine flexible sigmoidoscopy; 5–8 might be undertaken in a session.

Diagnostic and therapeutic colonoscopy There should be a maximum of six colonoscopies per session of one NHD.

Diagnostic and therapeutic endoscopic retrograde cholangiopancreatography (ERCP) A maximum of five procedures should be carried out in a session of one NHD.

On-call for gastroenterological emergencies

Sessional time will need to be allocated for an emergency out-of-hours endoscopy service.

Note. When there is training in endoscopic sessions, fewer patients can be seen.

Nutrition service

Consultant physicians with an interest in gastroenterology are usually responsible for leading the enteral and parenteral feeding service. Supervision of home-based parenteral nutrition is usually provided from specialist centres.

B Acute medicine *(see above)*

C Academic medicine

The clinical contribution of academic gastroenterologists varies widely, depending on their contract and other responsibilities.

2   Work to maintain and improve the quality of care

This work encompasses duties in clinical governance, professional self-regulation, continuing professional development, education and training of others. For many consultants, at various times in their careers, it may include research, serving in management, and providing advice. All require consultant participation. Such work is described fully in Part 1 of this document. Its scope is summarised in the Appendix to Part 2. Management and advisory work are identified specifically in the Appendix.

WORK PROGRAMME

Table 1 summarises an example of the work programme of consultant physicians undertaking gastroenterology and acute general medicine, giving the recommended workload, and allocation of notional half days (NHDs).

Table 1. Example of the work programme of a consultant physician in gastroenterology and general medicine, as notional half days (NHDs) per week

Activity	Workload	NHDs
Direct patient care		
Ward rounds and other inpatient work (except post-take rounds — see below)	2	2–3
Referrals	0–1	
Outpatient clinics		1–2
New patients	6–8 patients per clinic	
Follow-up patients		
General medical	15–20 patients per clinic	
Specialist	15–20 patients per clinic	

continued over

Diagnostic and therapeutic endoscopy		2
Diagnostic upper GI endoscopy	10–15 patients per clinic	
Therapeutic upper GI endoscopy	5–8 patients per clinic	
Diagnostic flexible sigmoidoscopy	10–15 patients per clinic	
Therapeutic flexible sigmoidoscopy	5–8 patients per clinic	
Diagnostic and therapeutic colonoscopy	6 patients per clinic	
Diagnostic and therapeutic ERCP	5 patients per clinic	
Nutrition service (usually in a specialist unit) Monitoring service	}	0–1

On-take, and mandatory post-take rounds	According to:
	  Numbers of admissions
	  Rota
	  Non-consultant support
		1–4

On-call for emergency endoscopy		0–1
Work to maintain and improve the quality of care		**3–5**

Total: The number of sessions worked by a consultant can be very variable. Most work programmes indicate an excess of 10 units worked. Obviously, there will be times in the career of a consultant when management and national duties will be carried out to increase the number of sessions.

WORKFORCE REQUIREMENTS FOR GASTROENTEROLOGY

i   Consultant NHDs required to provide a service in gastroenterology to a population of 250,000

The consultant requirement, measured as the number of consultant NHDs needed to provide a service, depends on the volume of inpatient, outpatient and endoscopic work, and can be calculated for any given workload. This paper gives a calculation of the consultant NHDs required to service the average workload of a district general hospital serving a population of 250,000. Although it is not yet universal practice, it is assumed that consultant physicians with an interest in gastroenterology work together to run a single inpatient service.

Inpatient service   Three consultant NHDs per week should be allocated for inpatient rounds, discharge letters and other related administration, with an additional consultant NHD per week for a post-take ward round.

Outpatient service   Outpatient services are often provided by the consultant staff and team in training. The reduction of junior doctors' hours and the commitment to run the emergency medical service often means that the junior medical staff cannot attend outpatient clinics regularly. In this example we have assumed that the consultant physician is working alone in outpatients.

New outpatient referrals   A district general hospital serving a population of 250,000 should see at least 4,100 new GI patients each year, including approximately 3,600 urgent cancer referrals as estimated in the 2-week cancer referral guidelines. (See appendix which gives the official estimates per 200,000) plus about 500 additional G-I and hepatology cases. A variable proportion of this workload, averaging about 1,500 cases, will be seen by gastrointestinal surgeons leaving about 2,600 cases. This requires eight to ten consultant NHDs weekly for consultants working alone in the outpatient clinic.

General medical outpatient follow-up post-discharge Up to two consultant NHDs are required weekly to provide this service.

Outpatient specialist follow up clinic per week Two consultant NHDs per week are required for this service.

Diagnostic and therapeutic endoscopy service

i. Diagnostic upper GI endoscopy and flexible sigmoidoscopy.

   The requirement for upper GI endoscopy in the general population is 1.5:100 population per annum. This gives an annual workload of 3,750 examinations in a district general hospital serving a population of 250,000. On the conservative assumption that at least two-thirds of lower GI urgent cancer referrals will require flexible sigmoidoscopy or colonoscopy, the requirement for flexible sigmoidoscopy gives a workload of 2/3 x 2,375 = 1,500 examinations per year of which 900 are likely to be provided by G-I physicians. Therefore, seven to nine NHDs per week are required for these procedures.

ii. Diagnostic and therapeutic colonoscopy and ERCP.

   Workload figures for the average district general hospital suggest that at least two NHDs per week are needed for diagnostic and therapeutic colonoscopy. One NHD is needed for diagnostic and therapeutic ERCP.

Out-of-hours endoscopy service This service requires up to one consultant NHD per week.

Nutrition service This service could add up to two consultant NHDs per week.

Monitoring service This service could add up to one consultant NHD per week.

Summary

Consultant NHDs required per week to provide a service in gastroenterology and general internal medicine in a DGH with an average workload.

Direct patient care

Where junior medical staff provide support for the inpatient service and consultants provide the outpatient and endoscopic service, about **38 NHDs** are required. The number of NHDs required to run the service is reduced if part of the work is undertaken by consultant colleagues and medical staff in training. For example, consultant colleagues in radiology or surgery might share the endoscopic workload. Regular help in outpatients by junior medical staff, each of whom might contribute to the work done by around 50% of that recommended for a consultant NHD, will also reduce that consultant sessional requirement. It should be noted that commitments may change with the development of outreach clinics in primary care and endoscopic services outside the specialist centres.

Work to maintain and improve the quality of care

Additional NHDs for each consultant are required for this work. Time must be allocated for each consultant for continuing medical education (CME) (1 NHD per week); teaching junior medical staff, nursing staff, and medical students (1NHD per week); administration and management (1NHD per week); and clinical research (1NHD per week).

On the basis of these conditions and recommendations the number of NHDs required by a District General Hospital serving a population of 250,000 to provide a clinical service in gastroenterology and general medicine can be calculated. Allowing 4 NHDs for each consultant for the supporting activities given above, the total is 61 NHDs.

Table 2 summarises the work programme of consultant gastroenterologists providing a service for a population of 250,000, giving the recommended workload, and allocation of notional half days (NHDs).

TABLE 2. The work of consultant gastroenterologists generated by a population of 250,000 (as notional half days (NHDs) per week).

Activity	Workload	NHDs per week for 250,000 population
Direct patient care		
Ward rounds (except on-take and post-take)		4
Outpatient clinics		
New patients	6–8 patients per clinic	8–10
Follow-up patients		
General medical	15–20 patients per clinic	2
Specialist	15–20 patients per clinic	2
		12–14
Diagnostic and therapeutic endoscopy		
Diagnostic upper GI endoscopy	10–15 patients per clinic	3,750 pa 5–7
Therapeutic upper GI endoscopy	5–8 patients per clinic	
Diagnostic flexible sigmoidoscopy	10–15 patients per clinic	1,000 pa 2
Therapeutic flexible sigmoidoscopy	5–8 patients per clinic	
Diagnostic and therapeutic colonoscopy	6 patients per clinic	2–3
Diagnostic and therapeutic ERCP	5 patients per clinic	1
		10–13
Nutrition service (usually in a specialist unit)		2–3
Monitoring service		
On-take, and mandatory post-take rounds	Rota 1:5 for this example	2–3
On-call for emergency endoscopy *(assuming some registrar input to the rota)*		4
Total direct patient care		34–41
Work to maintain and improve the quality of care (6 consultants)		24
Total		58–65

ii Consultant workforce requirement nationally

The calculation given above allows an estimate of the consultant requirement to be made. Assuming that teaching hospitals serve a population 13,478,000 and non-teaching hospitals a population of 38,251,000, the total need in England and Wales is for 1,310 whole-time consultants in gastroenterology (with general medicine). Currently there are 544. The National Cancer Plan (2000) states that 208 additional consultant posts would be provided over the next six years but even this increase leaves a major shortfall.

These calculations do not take into account an increasing demand for colorectal screening for cancer, already introduced for high risk individuals. It has been estimated that introduction of a screening programme for individuals who are not at increased risk would generate a requirement for an additional 160 consultants.

Editors note: *In 1999 there was insufficient information available to allow a more precise estimate of the workforce requirements in this specialty. This recent estimate provides a firmer basis for workforce planning but this too will need to be reviewed in the light of developments in practice and service delivery.*

Genitourinary medicine

i   The specialty and the clinical needs of the patients

Genitourinary medicine is outpatient based. The largest group of patients are those with sexually transmitted infections (STIs) such as gonorrhoea, syphilis, chlamydia and wart virus infection, and a wide range of allied conditions including, for example, erectile dysfunction. Close collaboration is needed with other specialties and supporting services, so clinics should be sited in acute general hospitals. The numbers of cases attending genitourinary medicine clinics have been rising in recent years and for the first time in 1998 over one million new diagnoses were made at clinics in England.[1] These increases have affected all STIs, with outbreaks reported from various parts of England.[2] Management of STIs is important in the control of human immunodeficiency virus (HIV) infection. Epidemiological evidence indicates that STIs predispose to the transmission of the virus[3] and this is supported by reports of increased viral load in infected genital secretions.[4] Failure to treat STIs in the early stages can lead to chronic complications such as pelvic inflammatory disease.

The other patients managed in genitourinary medicine are those with HIV infection. They form a smaller but more time-consuming group who develop a wide variety of medical, social and other problems. They also provide the inpatient component of genitourinary medicine. Their management involves multidisciplinary care in hospital and multiagency working between hospital and the community. The number of new HIV infections reported in the UK continues to increase[5] and the introduction of highly active anti-retroviral therapy (HAART) with multiple drugs has improved survival.[6] Therefore more patients require care.

ii   Organisation of the service at primary, secondary and tertiary levels

Primary care

An unknown number of patients are managed in primary care, but there is evidence of increased screening for *Chlamydia trachomatis* and referral to genitourinary medicine clinics.[7] This follows the Report of the CMO's Expert Advisory Group on *Chlamydia trachomatis*, which recommended community-based screening.[8] It is expected that the Sexual Health Strategy, prepared by the Department of Health, will emphasise management in primary care with increased screening and referral to genitourinary medicine clinics. The strategy will set standards for those providing care at this level, and genitourinary medicine will collaborate in developing protocols and training.

Secondary care

Genitourinary medicine specialists provide a hospital-based service in genitourinary medicine departments. There should be facilities for outpatients, and any service with HIV infected patients should have access to day care and beds. Although consultants work primarily in outpatient clinics, they provide on-call for urgent problems and support for other specialists. At least two consultants with appropriate supporting staff are required for a hospital serving a population of 250,000. It is essential that they have regular meetings with genitourinary medicine colleagues from surrounding units for audit and CPD.

Tertiary care

This is provided in genitourinary medicine clinics by specialists with special skills and training. Examples include sexual problems and vulval disorders. The Sexual Health Strategy may recommend the development of clinical networks, as in cancer care, to manage HIV infection. This will increase tertiary care.

iii Patterns of referral

Patients are free to attend genitourinary medicine clinics without referral from another provider. Historically clinics provided an open access walk-in facility. Recently the numbers of patients – and limited resources – have led to increased use of appointment systems. Patients still attend the clinic of their choice. This may or may not be near where they live or work because of travel or concerns about confidentiality. A small proportion are referred from general practice, family planning, accident and emergency departments and other providers.

Patients with HIV infection may prefer to seek treatment at major centres in conurbations. This pattern of care was facilitated by the principle that funding should follow patients. Currently the NHS is moving to district of residence based funding for STIs and HIV infection and this will encourage care within the district of residence. Referral patterns may be affected by clinical networks for HIV infected patients.

iv Ways of working, clinical networks and community arrangements

Most patients with STIs and allied conditions are managed within the clinics. A few patients require additional resources. For example, those with pelvic inflammatory disease and infertility require referral to other specialists. Genitourinary medicine clinics collaborate when caring for patients who travel, undertaking partner notification, or recalling patients failing to attend for follow-up, and they maintain informal networks for this purpose.

HIV-infected patients require integrated care, including joint care between hospital and general practice. This requires collaboration between primary care and secondary care and community health services such as nursing, social services and voluntary agencies.

v Characteristics of a high quality service

Service for sexually transmitted infections

- Patient suspecting an acute STI should be seen on the day they present to a clinic, or on the next occasion the clinic is open.[9] Most departments hold clinics at least four days per week and should have dedicated premises.
- Clinics should be in good quality easily accessible premises. There should be a relaxed atmosphere to assist confidential discussion of sexually related conditions. Interviewing rooms should be sound attenuated and examination rooms should afford privacy.[10]
- Management includes taking a general and sexual history, physical examination, and the collection of all appropriate specimens for a full STI screen.
- Clinical examination is supported by immediate staining and microscopy of samples, and patients are given results before leaving. This means the provision of fresh stains, swabs and other supplies, up to date and well-maintained equipment such as microscopes, and facilities for the storage and swift transfer of samples to arrive in the laboratories in optimal condition for processing.

continued over

▌ Patients often have more than one infection at one time. STIs may be asymptomatic so patients are offered screening for the common conditions.

▌ Provision of free treatment for STIs is a legal requirement[11] so treatments are stored and dispensed in the clinic.

▌ Patients with STIs are advised on the need to notify sexual partners at risk of infection, and they are offered counselling on sexual health in general. They are offered leaflets to support verbal information. They are also offered free condoms. Some clinics provide general contraceptive advice and all collaborate closely with related services.

▌ Follow-up appointments are required to assess resolution of symptoms and compliance with medication, undertake tests of cure, ensure partners have been notified, and for further sexual health advice if required.

▌ To provide this service, the medical staff are supported by receptionists, nurses, and health advisors.

▌ Enhanced confidentiality for all clinic attenders is set out in statute[11,12] to shield their identity as well as diagnosis, and must be guaranteed by all members of clinic staff and any other person who becomes aware of their attendance.

▌ All patients presenting to genitourinary medicine clinics are offered screening for HIV infection. This involves a discussion about the tests and the infection, which can be time-consuming for individuals with high-risk behaviour.

▌ The contracting process should ensure that this guidance is followed.[13–16]

Service for HIV infection

▌ A patient newly diagnosed with HIV infection should have an appointment for initial assessment within a week.

▌ At the first visit a full history is taken, physical examination performed, and an STI screen is offered if not previously done.

▌ Baseline investigations include viral load and CD4 lymphocyte subset, and those for co-existent or previous infection including tuberculosis if indicated. At this visit the patient may wish for further counselling.

▌ Though treatment may not be indicated at this stage, the services and facilities are described. These include the provision of anti-viral therapy (HAART), as well as drugs for prophylaxis or treatment of complications.[14] There may be a pharmacist on the spot to assist.

▌ There are advantages in dietitians, physiotherapists, and pharmacists taking part in all aspects of care, and patients should have access to community services and patient support groups.

▌ Patients require regular outpatient follow-up with monitoring of immunological and virological parameters. When these investigations indicate the need or symptoms develop, HAART will be introduced.

▌ When complications occur patients require outpatient, day centre or inpatient care in dedicated beds staffed by specially trained nurses. The clinical teams of outpatient-based doctors may manage all the hospital care supported in outpatients and the day centre primarily by nurses.

▌ High quality care requires close cooperation and good communication between all those involved in the wards, outpatients and the community.

▌ Longer appointment times are required for these patients than those with STI.

▌ The contracting process should ensure that this guidance is followed.

vi   Outline of clinical work of consultants in genitourinary medicine

Consultants undertake five or six sessions every week in the outpatient clinic seeing STI and HIV infected patients, and one or two sessions in the wards. The work varies depending on local needs, overall service provision and the particular skills and experience of individuals. Some consultants concentrate on HIV infected patients whilst others see few or none. Consultants with special skills and training may work in psychosexual and vulval clinics, clinics for lipid [**DN Is this correct?**] disorders, and mother and baby HIV sessions, for example.

Consultants supervise inpatient care, sometimes shared with colleagues in other disciplines, with two ward rounds a week taking one or two sessions. They may also supervise or share in hospice care for HIV infected patients. Genitourinary medicine consultants seldom visit patients in other hospitals or undertake domiciliary visits.

Many consultants work in more than one hospital. They may be on-call for emergencies at several hospitals. Time must be allowed for travel and car-parking space might be essential. Some consultants undertake this work without any supporting medical staff. Others based at a single hospital with colleagues and good supporting staff have less onerous on-call commitments.

vii   Outline of the work of other members of the team

In STI clinics the following are the main groups of staff.

Doctors

- Consultants are supported by NCCGs, specialist registrars and SHOs.
- The doctors take the history and undertake clinical examination of all new patients.
- They tell the patients their diagnoses, prescribe and may dispense treatment.
- In small clinics they may collect the samples, undertake microscopy, advise on partner notification, undertake counselling and arrange follow-up appointments.

Nurses

- Nurses are trained to take samples for investigation, and undertake microscopy.
- They help with partner notification and counselling.
- They dispense prescribed treatment according to agreed written guidelines. This may include treatment of warts.
- In HIV clinics they must be familiar with the wide range of clinical and other problems that arise. They are trained to assist with or to undertake a wide range of procedures such as obtaining induced sputum samples, intravenous infusions and biopsies. They need to know, and may liaise with, services in the hospital and community.
- Nurse practitioners undertake independent practice according to agreed written guidelines.

Health advisors

Health advisors are professionals unique to genitourinary medicine. All clinics have one or more on duty throughout all clinic sessions. They have three main roles.

- Advise patients on notifying partners at risk of infection. This involves identifying the individuals and working with the patient to determine the best way of to ensure attendance at a clinic. It may include talking to the partner on behalf of the patient.

- Provide the main counselling service in clinics. All patients are anxious about their attendance at a clinic, their diagnosis, treatment and sequelae. Patients whose behaviour has put them at risk of acquiring HIV infection may require much discussion before and after antibody testing. This may include on-going support of HIV infected patients.

- Ensure attendance of patients for review to assess response to treatment. This is a vital part of infection control, especially with the rising incidence of STIs and HIV infection.

Receptionists

These staff have a difficult role. They have the first contact with new patients who are occasionally aggressive. For reasons of confidentiality and because patients may attend without appointments, clinics have their own dedicated healthcare records for which receptionists are responsible.

Other staff

These include clinical psychologists, psychosexual counsellors, pharmacists and dietitians.

viii Conjoined services

- High quality clinical microbiological and virology laboratories.

- On the spot imaging. Routine radiology should be supplemented by ultrasound, CT scans, MRI and radio-nucleotide imaging where possible.

- Later stages of HIV infection require close collaboration between many hospital specialists and between secondary care, primary care and community nursing, dietetics, midwifery, home helps, residential and hospice care, and voluntary organisations.

ix Specialised facilities required

- Modern tilting couches for the examination of female and disabled patients.

- Supplies and equipment for on the spot microscopy.

- Facilities for collecting, storing and transporting samples to the laboratories.

- Equipment for the treatment of warts which may include cryotherapy and electrocautery by means of a hyfrecator; access to laser therapy is an advantage. Some specialists undertake colposcopy.

- Stand alone computer systems for clinical data including the patient index; for reasons of confidentiality these systems should not be connected to main hospital networks.

- Computer links with supporting investigation departments to facilitate rapid report and results services; these must use coded identifiers and strict password protected access.

- HIV infected cases require a range of facilities including arterial puncture for blood gases, lung function tests, negative pressure rooms for obtaining induced sputum and for admission if pulmonary tuberculosis and other aerosol infections are present or suspected, and day care for treatment such as intermittent iv infusions.

x   **Quality**

See sections v, vi and references 9, 10, 13–14.

The UK national guidelines for the management of STIs are under revision by the genitourinary medicine Clinical Effectiveness Group, which keeps in close touch with the College on the format to be adopted.

Consultants review the notes of all patients to monitor quality of care and ensure that accurate diagnoses are entered on returns. (Workload and epidemiological returns are made to Trusts, districts, regions, and to the PHLS on behalf of the Department of Health.)

Genitourinary medicine clinics undertake internal and multidisciplinary audits, for example, in-clinic microscopy results are audited against laboratory results. Most regions have a well developed system of regional audits which are reported to the NHSE Regional Offices.

xi   **Contribution to acute medicine**

Few genitourinary medicine physicians participate in general medical take but they do provide a consultation service, including out-of-hours provision.

xii   **Academic physicians**

Academic genitourinary physicians undertake similar clinical NHS duties to NHS consultants according to agreed job plans. They make a strong contribution to the NHS. Major advances have followed collaboration between clinicians and scientists.

xiii   **Improving patient care**

Though the new Sexual Health Strategy will probably emphasise more community based care and set standards for this, it is anticipated that the overall effect will be to increase patient attendance at clinics. The main requirement for improved patient care is adequate resource.

The prime need is to be able to see patients suspecting new STIs either on the day they present or on the next occasion the clinic is open.[9] Whether this is best provided by open access or flexible appointment systems needs to be determined. Thought also needs to be given to more early morning, late evening and weekend working but these will need adequate resource. Staff skill mix and multidisciplinary working requires more consideration. Discussion is needed within the specialty, with purchasers and with the DoH to introduce these improvements.

Improved laboratory diagnosis is required including the wide introduction of sensitive methods for detecting microrganisms, such as DNA amplification, and improved antimicrobial sensitivity testing. Though DNA amplification tests are more expensive than current methods, the technology is available to undertake tests for multiple organisms on single samples at little more cost than a single investigation. Another improvement will be salivary antibody detection instead of serological testing. Implicit in these developments is the need to produce timely reports. Introducing these will require co-operation in trusts between laboratories and clinics, more widely between the PHLS and trusts, and may benefit from discussion between the RCP and RCPath.

Improved computer systems within clinics are required, especially if disaggregated workload and epidemiological data are collected; currently summed data are collected. The more complex disaggregated data collection is under debate. Clinical networking will also require better systems. Improvement will require work with industry; while the RCP Genitourinary Medicine Liaison Committee can provide an impetus, probably the Association for Genitourinary Medicine will need to facilitate these changes.

Treatment of HIV infection needs antiretrovirals with enhanced potency and simpler dosing regimens. Many clinics are currently working with the MRC and industry in developing drugs.

The specialty has good treatment and service guidelines.[13–14] These have been taken forward by the genitourinary medicine Clinical Effectiveness Group, the Association for Genitourinary Medicine and the British HIV Association. Whilst most clinical care is covered by these guidelines, services should have agreed written guidance for all aspects of management. This will improve and maintain quality and maximise risk avoidance and risk management.

The specialty is working on a document which outlines the application of clinical governance in genitourinary medicine. This can made available to the College when it is finished.

WORK OF CONSULTANTS IN GENITOURINARY MEDICINE

1 Direct patient care

A Work in the specialty

Inpatient work

This largely concerns HIV-infected patients. Many services have a policy of managing most care on an outpatient basis. Admissions are mainly emergencies. A few patients may be admitted for procedures such as endoscopy or insertion of a permanent iv line.

Ward rounds These vary according to the numbers of patients involved and the supporting staff available. Many DGHs have only one or two inpatients at any one time. Consultants in DGHs may be single handed with minimal supporting staff. They may see the patients daily and manage all or most of the care themselves. Alternatively, inpatient care may be shared with colleagues in other disciplines such as infection or thoracic medicine with shared junior staff.

Larger units have several genitourinary medicine consultants with either dedicated or shared junior staff. Regular ward rounds, which provide an opportunity for clinical teaching, take place, preferably with the full team of junior medical staff, specialist nurses, pharmacists, physiotherapists, dietitians and others.

Referral work Consultants in genitourinary medicine swiftly see referrals from other wards, for example when HIV infected patients are admitted to other services.

Interspecialty, interdisciplinary liaison and case conferences

Services with many HIV infected inpatients hold a regular weekly clinical meeting or round attended by clinicians from all disciplines involved, where all inpatients and problem outpatients are discussed. Clinicians from the investigation departments make useful contributions. Other providers such as pharmacists, dietitians, physiotherapists and clinical psychologists attend. If regular meetings cannot be held, there should be alternative arrangements to serve a similar purpose. These meetings have an important training role.

A single-handed consultant should only manage occasional inpatients. A team of five consultants can manage 10 to 20 inpatients with rotations for on-call and day-to-day consultant supervision.

Outpatient clinics

STI clinics   Most departments hold clinics on at least four days per week. The specialty believes that in an NHS moving towards a consultant based service, genitourinary medicine should aim for consultants seeing 50% or more of patients. In a $3\frac{1}{2}$ hour session consultants should allow 3 hours for their own patients and $\frac{1}{2}$ hour for consultation, teaching and training. Clinical teaching forms an essential part of the workload in teaching and non-teaching hospitals. In an STI clinic a consultant can see 4 to 6 new patients and 8 to 12 for review. Numbers vary according to the case mix, and the supporting staff. Adequate time must be allowed to practise to a satisfactory standard; this is especially important for single-handed consultants.

Purchasers and trusts may require late evening and early morning or weekend clinics which must be staffed in the same manner as other sessions.

HIV clinics   Consultants seeing HIV infected patients require the support of junior medical staff who need additional training. There should also be receptionists, nurses and health advisors. Ideally, where dedicated HIV clinics are held, other healthcare professionals should be available including pharmacists, dietitians and clinical psychologists. A consultant should see 5–9 patients in a 3-hour session.

Other specialist clinics   Consultants may undertake other clinics depending on case mix and local requirements. These may include psychosexual problems and erectile dysfunction, and clinical problem clinics such as pelvic pain. These require nursing support. Some services provide multidisciplinary clinics such as those for genital skin or vulval disorders staffed by a genitourinary medicine physician, dermatologist and gynaecologist, who see the patients together. These clinics provide opportunities for teaching and training. Six to nine patients can be seen in a 3-hour session.

Specialised investigative and therapeutic procedure clinics

Investigative clinics   For some years genitourinary medicine provided colposcopy, but with the increasing pressures of other work this service is being reduced. Colposcopy is needed for vulval clinics.

Therapeutic procedure clinics   Genital warts are common and persistent. They can be treated in dedicated sessions or during dedicated time. Trained nurses working to written agreed protocols may provide treatment. One person using one room can treat 4–6 patients per hour. Intermittent intravenous infusions and inhalation therapy are provided as required.

Specialised services within the specialty   These include no need for referral from another provider, ease of access, confidentiality of identity and diagnosis, clinical diagnosis supported by on the spot microscopy, swift systems for transferring samples to supporting laboratories, and free treatment.

In addition there is sexual health counselling including contraception and provision of free condoms, discussion of HIV antibody testing, partner notification, management of erectile dysfunction, joint management of genital dermatoses and vulval disorders, and, in some services, colposcopy. Most services provide HIV infection outpatient care and many provide the medical element of full HIV care.

Services outwith the base hospital   Many consultants work at more that one hospital. Adequate travel time and car parking are required. A few consultants with large HIV workloads visit patients in hospices either to supervise or share in their care. Currently few genitourinary medicine services undertake outreach clinics, largely because of the difficulties associated with confidentiality, the need for on the spot microscopy and for readily available investigative support.

On-call for specialist advice   All services provide a consultant on call. This includes advice on HIV post-exposure prophylaxis following needlestick injuries, support for A&E departments, inpatients, and sometimes problems in the community. With aid of junior staff some emergencies may be managed over the telephone or using other telemedicine modes. Some single-handed consultants still have 1 in 1 rotas at more than one hospital.

B Acute medicine

Consultants in genitourinary medicine do not participate in the on-take rota for unselected medical emergencies.

C Academic medicine

See section xii above.

2   Work to maintain and improve the quality of care

This work encompasses duties in clinical governance, professional self-regulation, continuing professional development, education and training of others. For many consultants, at various times in their careers, it may include research, serving in management, and providing advice. All require consultant participation. Such work is described fully in Part 1 of this document. Its scope is summarised in the Appendix to Part 2. Management and advisory work are identified specifically in the Appendix.

Summary of the time spent on the various duties required of a consultant

Activity	NHDs
Direct patient care	
Outpatient clinics including HIV care (fixed)	5–6
Ward work including day care (fixed)	$1/_2$–2
On call	$1/_2$–2
Work to maintain and improve the quality of care	
Clinical governance, including audit	$1/_2$
Professional regulation including CPD and contributing to development of clinical standards	1
Education and training	$1/_2$–1
Research	0–1
Management and advice including committee work	1

WORKFORCE REQUIREMENTS FOR GENITOURINARY MEDICINE

The specialty returns the number of patient visits to trusts, districts, regions, and to the PHLS on behalf of the Department of Health (of which there were 1,614,060 in 1998–99) and has undertaken surveys to determine average patient consultation times. Recent surveys, including one commissioned by the Department of Health, indicate that the service is not adequate to meet the patient need. Currently consultants see about 30% of outpatients. As the NHS is moving towards a consultant based service the specialty believes consultants should see 50% or more of patients.

Calculations

Consultants in genitourinary medicine required (WTE) for a hospital serving a population of 250,000

The consultant workforce requirement has been calculated for a hospital serving a population of 250,000. It is based on the number of consultations in 1998–99, with consultants seeing 50% of cases, spending 3 hours of each NHD seeing patients, and working 42 weeks of the year. Surveys have shown that the mean number of consultations for new and review cases of sexually transmitted infection (STI) is 4.1 per hour; and for new and review cases of HIV infections is 2 per hour.

Consultations in genitourinary medicine required by a population of 250,000

1. *Average number of STI consultations per year*

New	3,496
Review	5,704
Total	*9,200*

With a mean number of 4.1 consultations per hour, a 3-hour session (NHD) provides for 12.3 consultations. Therefore 748 sessions are required for 9,200 consultations.

2. *Average number of HIV consultations per year*

New	92
Review	151
Total	*243*

With a mean number of two consultations per hour, a 3-hour session (NHD) provides for six consultations. Therefore 40.5 sessions are required for 243 HIV consultations.

Thus a total of 991 sessions (NHDs) are required on average for a population of 250,000.

A consultant provides 420 sessions (NHDs) per year, of which 42 are for inpatients and 84–168 (2–4 per week) – say 126 – are allocated to work to maintain and improve the quality of care. This leaves about 294 for STI outpatient work.

If consultants see 50% of all cases, the total number of consultant outpatient sessions (NHDs) required for STI and HIV consultations is 394. An uplift of 100 sessions (100 NHDs) is made for underprovision, together with 1 session per week (52 NHDs) for inpatient and on-call work. The total is 546 sessions (NHDs) per year. This is equivalent to 2.1 WTE consultants, or 1 per 120,000 of the population.

Large local populations generate more STIs and HIV cases than small ones, so nationally based estimates are more accurate than the local ones. The hospital figures support the principle that single-handed posts are unsatisfactory. The figures assume that all consultants have adequate support of junior medical and other staff.

Currently the numbers of patients attending clinics are increasing.[1] Real increases in most infections have been observed over the last few years. In addition there has been increasing screening for C trachomatis in the community with many infected patients referred to clinics for management.[7] It is thought likely that the recommendations of the Sexual Health Strategy will increase awareness leading to more patients. It is probable that the workforce estimates will need to be revised upwards.

National workforce requirements

At present there are 231 WTE consultants for a population of ca 51.7 million in England, Wales and Northern Ireland. They see about 30% of the patients. If consultants were to see 50% of outpatients, which would require 2.1 consultants per 250,000 population, the total number (WTE) of consultants in genitourinary medicine required nationally is 435. There is a shortfall of 204 (or 88%).

NOTE: *In 1999 there was insufficient information available to allow a more precise estimate of the workforce requirements in this specialty. This recent estimate provides a firmer basis for workforce planning but this too will need to be reviewed in the light of developments in practice and service delivery.*

References

1. PHLS, DHSS, and PS, Scottish IS(D)5 Collaborative Group. *Trends in sexually transmitted infections in the United Kingdom 1990–1999.* London: Public Health Laboratory Service, 2000.

2. Outbreak of heterosexually acquired syphilis in Cambridgeshire. *Commun Dis Rep CDR Wkly* 2000;**10**:401.

3. Fleming DT, Wasserheit JN. From epidemiological synergy to public health policy and practice: the contribution of other sexually transmitted diseases to sexual transmission of HIV infection. *Sex Transm Inf* 1999;**75**:3–17.

4. Moss GB, Overbaugh J, Welch M *et al.* Human immunodeficiency virus DNA in urethral secretions in men: association with gonococcal urethritis and CD4 depletion. *J Infect Dis* 1995;**172**:1469–74.

5. AIDS and HIV infection in the United Kingdom: monthly report. http://www.phls.co.uk/publications/CDRelectronic/CDR%20weekly/CDR%20.../hiv.htm2001. 29/01/2001.

6. Rogers PA, Sinka KJ, Molesworth AM *et al.* Survival after diagnosis of AIDS among adults resident in the United Kingdom in the era of multiple therapies. *Commun Dis Public Health* 2000;**3**:188–94.

7. Evans DTP. Comparative sources of positive female chlamydia diagnoses and places of treatment of chlamydia in Leicester 1997–1999 inclusive. A changing trend? *Int J STD & AIDS* 2001;**12**:62.

8. Report of CMOs advisory group on Chlamydia trachomatis. London: Department of Health, 1998.

9. Report of the working party to examine work loads in genitourinary medicine (the 'Monks Report'). London: Department of Health, 1988.

10. Health Building Note 12, Supplement 1, Genitourinary medicine clinics, Department of Health, Welsh Office. Department of Health (NI), 1990.

11. The Public Health (Venereal Diseases) Regulations 1916. Ministry of Health, London.

12. The National Health Service (Venereal Diseases) Regulations 1974. Department of Health and Social Security, London.

13. *Guidelines for a GU medicine service specification.* Association for Genitourinary Medicine, 1995.

14. Service standards in genitourinary medicine; advisory document for purchaser/clinical governance leads. Association for Genitourinary Medicine, 2000.

15. Considerations for core service specification. Association for Genitourinary Medicine, 2000.

16. Radcliffe K, Ahmad-Jushuf I, Cowan F *et al.* UK national guidelines on sexually transmitted infections and closely allied conditions. *Sex Transm Infect* 1999;**75**:Supplement 1.

17. *Guidelines for the management of HIV infection in the UK.* British HIV Association, 2000.

Geriatric medicine

i   A brief description of the specialty and the clinical needs of patients

The essence of geriatric medicine as a specialty is to assess and treat the medical and rehabilitative needs of older people. This is done through a process known as comprehensive geriatric assessment (CGA). There is a body of evidence which shows that the outcomes for older people with multiple pathologies and functional problems are better if they have their treatment overseen by an interdisciplinary team (see Box 1) led by a consultant specialist in geriatric medicine.[1,2]

Thus, depending on the nature of the illness and the degree of disability, the core work of a geriatric medical service may take place in a number of different inpatient areas. These include emergency treatment of older people within the general hospital. This is frequently followed by an intensive period of rehabilitation after the acute illness, both in the general hospital and in less acute settings such as community hospitals, through the utilisation of the skills of the multidisciplinary team to improve or maintain physical function in the face of illness. For a small number of patients, with ongoing requirements for specialist review, there will be a need for continuing care.[3]

Most geriatric services also have community services, including outpatients, community outreach teams, and day hospital facilities. These services aim to support older people in the community who require specialist medical supervision of their medical condition and at times improvement or maintenance of their physical function.

In addition, some units have structured services for orthogeriatrics, movement disorders, and stroke (of which the last two may be services for patients of any age). Whilst such specialised services are highly desirable, given current staffing levels they cannot be regarded as core services. In many parts of the country these services are absent or patchy.

ii   Organisation of the service

The acute inpatient assessment of older people needs to take place as soon as possible after the patient reaches hospital with an illness. Therefore, acute assessment facilities should be an integral component on the main hospital site close to all investigative facilities and other supporting specialties. Organisation of services must be geared towards this goal although the methodology may vary. As noted in the *National service framework for older people*,[4] there is no firm evidence for using any one particular format, ie integrated with general medicine, age related or needs related. Patients that are admitted urgently to geriatric medical services might be referred directly by their general practitioners, through medical admissions units or from other acute areas, especially orthopaedics.

Rehabilitation aims to restore or maintain physical function, eg walking or independence in dressing. This should be commenced as soon as the patient stabilises after an admission for acute illness within the general hospital. However, rehabilitation may take place in various settings, many of which are away from the main hospital site (in the proposed forms of intermediate care). These patients often have complex medico-social problems although they are not normally acutely unwell on admission. But most are frail and vulnerable, and become ill during admission. Such services need to be carefully planned and evaluated.[5,6]

Day hospitals form much of the focus of comprehensive geriatric assessment and rehabilitation reaching out into the community on an outpatient basis. Day hospitals have also become a hub of activity relating to some of the application of sub-specialist clinics mentioned above. The activity of the day hospital will depend on the availability of nursing, paramedical and medical staff as well as other local resources.

Although the number of NHS continuing care beds has been reduced, continuing care has actually increased, but is now scattered through a variety of institutions and organisations. Thus the role of the geriatrician is often to facilitate good practice through co-ordination of interdisciplinary outreach.

iii   Special patterns of referral

Geriatricians receive referrals from most hospital specialties, often through formal liaison, most often from general medicine, orthopaedics; general surgery and psychiatry of old age. In many services these responsibilities are split between the participating consultants, and a consultant would expect to receive 5–10 such referrals per week. A similar number of emergency referrals from primary care would be expected each week.

iv   Ways of working, clinical networks, community arrangements

Consultants in geriatric medicine pioneered the concept of interdisciplinary team working to ensure that both medical illness and functional capacity was assessed and treated in older people. Therefore, it is the essence of good practice in acute assessment and rehabilitation settings for the consultant to lead at least one interdisciplinary case conference per week. These may be less frequent in continuing care.

v   Describe the characteristics of a high quality service

Working within an ideal environment of adequate physical and personnel resources, the consultant specialist in geriatric medicine and their team should be able to offer:

- a comprehensive assessment of older patients' needs within 24 hours of admission with an acute illness and transfer to specialist beds on demand
- commencement of rehabilitation on the general hospital site as soon as possible after acute illness stabilises
- rehabilitation away from the general hospital site for patients who no longer require access to its investigative and support facilities
- inpatient continuing care for those with profound disability and on-going medical/nursing needs
- a series of formal liaison protocols with acute general medicine; orthopaedics, general surgery, and psychiatry of old age

▌ in co-operation with other medical specialists, a highly developed service for people who have suffered strokes, encompassing both fast-track outpatient investigation and inpatient assessment and rehabilitation

▌ a consultative service to primary care where patients needs are not acute, including formal outreach services as well as day hospital and outpatient services

▌ a variety of sub-specialist services including for example, movement disorders, orthogeriatrics and falls services.

vi Outline of clinical work in the specialty

The work of individual geriatricians differs widely, both in content and load, across the United Kingdom. This reflects variations in local supporting services, specialist activity, and geographical sites to be covered as well as involvement in acute work.

Most consultants in geriatric medicine will maintain specific sessional commitment to the inpatient core areas of acute assessment, rehabilitation, and continuing care. Additionally they will have some community responsibilities through outpatients, day hospital and outreach facilities. In well-staffed departments the responsibility for the common sub-specialisms of orthogeriatrics and stroke will divided between consultants. Other sub-specialist work geriatricians frequently undertake such as movement disorders, and cognitive dysfunction will often depend on local circumstances.

Many geriatricians now also incorporate organ sub-specialisms into their work. Local requirements and personal interests have often brought these about. Such specialisms include: diabetes, falls and osteoporosis, clinical pharmacology and heart failure.

The nature of geriatric medicine and its interaction with the community will often mean that services are provided off the main site. The development of intermediate or post acute care, in co-operation with primary care will tend to increase this area of work.

vii Work of the other members of the multidisciplinary team

The practice of geriatric medicine relies very heavily on collating information provided by various paramedical and medical specialties, much as other specialists might use pathology or radiodiagnostic imaging. Cases are discussed on a regular basis with the team members to arrive at an agreed treatment plan that is lead by the consultant. If there are deficiencies in personnel then it will be difficult for the team to ensure the full gains of comprehensive geriatric assessment.

viii Complementary services

The most specific complementary services are listed in Box 1. The unpredictable nature of illness in old age means that proximity to other mainstream specialists is a requirement.

Box 1: Medical and paramedical services required to support assessment and rehabilitation

Activities of daily living
Occupational therapy

Care management
Social work services

Communication
Speech and language therapy
Audiology
Hearing therapy
Ophthalmology
Optician
Dental Services

Elimination
Continence advisor
Stoma therapist
Urological/gynaecological services
Urodynamic assessment
Personal laundry services

Nutrition
Dietetics
Enteral and parenteral feeding services
Dental services

Mental state
Psychiatry of old age
Clinical psychology

Mobility
Physiotherapy
Wheelchair and aid supplies
Orthotics
Podiatry
Orthopaedic services

---

ix **Specialised facilities required**

Those units running stroke services will need to have access to specialised neuro-imaging, doppler scanning and swallowing assessments. Otherwise, it is essential that older patients have good gymnasium facilities for early rehabilitation and areas to perform adequate assessment of activities of daily living, eg occupational therapy bathrooms and kitchens.

x **Quality standards and measures of the quality of the specialised service**

Both the Health Advisory Service in England (HAS 2000) and the Scottish Health Advisory Service utilise quality indicators on their visits to services for older people. These include basic needs for physical fabric as well as standards concerning core and sub-specialty services and personnel requirements.

WORK OF CONSULTANTS IN GERIATRICS

1   Direct patient care

A Work in the specialty

Inpatient work

Acute inpatient care (see also section B below) Depending on case mix, number of beds and support staffing, a consultant would expect to perform at least two assessment ward rounds per week. A consultant should not normally be expected to care for more than 20 acutely ill assessment patients at any one time. It is anticipated that each consultant might receive between 5–10 acutely ill new specialty patients per week.
Time required: 2 NHD.

Rehabilitation A consultant, with supporting medical staff, should be expected to care for no more than 20 rehabilitation patients at any one time, with 200–300 discharges per year. A consultant would normally be expected to complete at least one rehabilitation ward round each week per 20 patients.
Time required: 1 NHD.

Continuing care A geriatrician should have direct responsibility for no more than 30 continuing care beds. A consultant would normally be expected to review patients at least every other week, with regular and comprehensive assessment their needs. It is also likely that patients will have all their medical requirements met in the unit and only rarely will there be a need for transfer.
Time required: 1 NHD, flexibly allocated.

Referral work A consultant would expect to deal with 5–10 referrals per week.

Inter-specialty and inter-disciplinary liaison
Time required: 1 NHD.

Case conferences
Time required: included in ward rounds.

Over and above these, considerable time is spent on speaking to carers and relatives to adequately consult and plan discharges.
Time required: 0.5 NHD.

Outpatient work

General geriatric medicine clinics

The number of patients who can be seen will depend on resources and will rise with the amount of support:

New patients:	2–4 when no support
Patients for review:	4–9 when no support

Specialised clinics within the specialty

Common sub-specialisms include:

▪ *Stroke and TIA clinics;* movement disorders and cognitive dysfunction.

The numbers of patients who can be seen and the time required depend on the amount of medical and other support.
Time required: As allocated.

▪ *Acute general medical clinic*
New patients
Follow-up patients

▪ *Non-acute general medical clinic*
New patients
Follow-up patients

The nature of the post and the amount of general medicine in the job will determine these figures.
Time required: 1 NHD per clinic.

Day hospitals

A high turnover day hospital might expect to see 600 new patients a year in a 30 placed unit. Each consultant should have no more than 12–15 patients each at any one time. The consultant can expect to personally review 30–50% of these patients and hold interdisciplinary case conferences on them every 1–2 weeks.
Time required: 1 NHD.

Services outwith the base hospital

▪ Clinics at other hospitals
▪ Outreach clinics
▪ Domiciliary work
▪ Hospice work.

Time required: 1 NHD per timetabled session.

On-call for specialist advice and emergencies

Geriatric medicine remains a major bed holding specialty, and most geriatricians provide on-call rotas in addition to other acute rota requirements (see section B below). The frequency of call-out and the intensity of work varies, depending on the amount of experienced non-consultant support.

On-call for specialist advice and emergency attendance:

SpR available	1 NHD each week
SHO available	2 NHDs each week
Rota more often than 1:4	an additional 0.5 NHD each week.

B Acute medicine

According to the RCP London manpower survey, approximately 70% of the geriatricians in England and Wales, who completed the survey questionnaire, have some input into unselected acute general medical take.[7] However, the absolute figure may be lower as the return rate was 70%. It is clear from the manpower returns that the nature of this acute activity is very variable. It should be noted that most physicians performing acute take duties should not have to take personal responsibility for more than 25 acute admissions per day. Where the geriatrician takes part in acute medical take they may find that it is difficult to reconcile this with other duties, which take them off the main site. This is particularly the case when they have little in the way of non-consultant support.

Emergency take and post-take rounds (see Part 1 of this volume).

C Academic medicine

Many academic departments of geriatric medicine are small and academic geriatricians often share patient care duties with NHS colleagues. They have a heavy burden of teaching not only of medical students but also of other disciplines, as well as the requirement for research and other academic duties. Clinical commitments are a matter of negotiation and are often arranged as part of a corporate departmental plan. Similarly, many NHS geriatricians shoulder a large burden of teaching and research where there is no academic department. Each consultant should have appropriate time allocated for teaching and research.

2 Work to maintain and improve the quality of care

This work encompasses duties in clinical governance, professional self-regulation, continuing professional development, education and training of others. For many consultants, at various times in their careers, it may include research, serving in management, and providing advice. All require consultant participation. Such work is described fully in Part 1 of this document. Its scope is summarised in the Appendix to Part 2. Management and advisory work are identified specifically in the Appendix.

The British Geriatrics Society has produced detailed guidance on clinical governance in the specialty and the amount of time that will be required to fulfil these requirements.[8]

Generally a lead clinician in clinical governance would need 1 NHD whilst participation would need approximately 0.25 NHD. This does not include any time required for revalidation or participation in appraisal.

WORKFORCE REQUIREMENTS FOR GERIATRICS

In 1997 there were 761 consultants, ie 1 per 70,171 of the population. Currently the minimum recommendation for the adequate provision of core services is 1 per 50,000 of the population; and, more appropriately, 1 per 4,000 of the population aged 75 or over. Where there are significant extra duties in general medicine or sub-specialisms such as stroke etc, then this figure should be modified. Other factors which should be taken in to account are teaching and research commitments, the geography of the area, the number of sites to be covered and the numbers and experience of supporting staff of all grades and specialisms.

The population is ageing, and it is recognised that there will be increasing time requirements with clinical governance and revalidation. There is a current academic personnel shortfall and the expectations of the National Service Framework will require greater community activity and assessment. Thus, it is believed that the minimum projected figure of 1,368 consultant geriatricians by 2009 for England and Wales (and allowing for part time working) will need to be re-evaluated.

NOTE: *In 1999 there was insufficient information available to allow a more precise estimate of the workforce requirements in this specialty. This recent estimate provides a firmer basis for workforce planning but this too will need to be reviewed in the light of developments in practice and service delivery.*

References

1. Stuck AE, Sui AL, Wieland GD, Adams J, Rubenstein LZ. Comprehensive geriatric assessment: a meta-analysis of controlled trials. *Lancet* 1993;**342**:1032–1036.

2. Audit Commission. *The way to go home: rehabilitation and remedial services for older people.* National report by the Audit Commission, 2000.

3. Royal College of Physicians of London. *Management of the older medical patient. Teamwork in the journey of care.* London: Royal College of Physicians, 2000.

4. Department of Health. *National service framework for older people.* London: Department of Health, 2001. www.doh.gov.uk/nsf/olderpeople.htm

5. *Rehabilitation of older people.* British Geriatrics Society, Compendium 2000. www.bgs.org.uk

6. *Intermediate care: guidance for commissioners and providers of health and social care.* British Geriatrics Society, Compendium 2000. www.bgs.org.uk

7. Royal College of Physicians. *Summary of information: consultant workforce in medical specialties in England, Wales and Northern Ireland, 1999.* London: Royal College of Physicians, 2000.

8. *Guidelines for the implementation of clinical governance in geriatric medicine.* Recommendations of the British Geriatrics Society and Royal Colleges of Physicians. British Geriatrics Society, Compendium. 2000. www.bgs.org.uk

Haematology

i Introduction

Haematology encompasses clinical management of blood disorders, laboratory measurement of cellular components of blood, provision and proper use of transfusion products, and laboratory identification and clinical management of disturbances in haemostasis. Haematologists undergo general professional training in medicine and specialist training in all aspects of haematology, both clinical and laboratory. Consultant haematologists are expected to maintain a core competence in both laboratory and clinical haematology, to provide an on-call and emergency service. However, most haematologists have further competences in one or more sub-specialties within the discipline. These sub-specialties are organised according to the special needs of groups of patients and include:

- Haemato-oncology: acute and chronic leukaemias, lymphoma, multiple myeloma
- Haemostasis/thrombosis: haemophilia, thrombophilia, acquired bleeding disorders
- Disorders of blood production and destruction: bone marrow failure, myeloproliferative disorders, myelodysplastic syndromes, inherited and acquired; haemolytic anaemias, autoimmune blood diseases, haemoglobinopathies
- Transfusion medicine: blood transfusion services; therapeutic apheresis
- Paediatric haematology.

Haematologists provide the medical professional input into the organisation of laboratories, interpretation of morphology and histology of haematological specimens, including immuno-phenotyping and cytochemistry, and an advisory service on haematological matters to other departments within a general hospital.

The clinical need

General haematology

Patients with all kinds of anaemia may present to a haematologist or be referred for specialist investigation. Acquired bleeding disorders in adults and children require referral to a haematologist. Specialist units in surgery, medicine and obstetrics, in a general hospital, all require haematological services to manage associated haematological problems, those of haemostasis and thrombosis, and transfusion.

Haemato-oncology

There are about 5,000 new cases of adult acute and chronic leukaemia each year in England and Wales.[1] About three-quarters occur in patients over the age of 50. Acute lymphoblastic leukaemia is most common in children and young adults. Patients of all ages may be affected by acute or chronic myeloid leukaemia. There are about 7,000 new cases of non-Hodgkin's lymphoma each year, the number having increased over the last 20 years, and two-thirds are in patients over the age of 60.[2] There are 1200 new cases of Hodgkin's disease each year, the majority of patients being less than 60 years old. Myeloma, which is more common over the age of 40, produces 3,000 new cases each year. Most require intensive chemotherapy and long-term follow-up. The prevalence of these diseases also increases with longer survival and better cure rates, with more patients requiring follow-up.

Genetic disorders

Several lifelong and inherited disorders, among them haemophilia, the haemoglobinopathies, thalassaemias and sickle cell disease, require care and management by haematologists.

ii Organisation

Primary care

The haematology laboratory provides the service for primary care, and the haematologist provides advisory and interpretative services to back up the laboratory results. The haematologist is an essential link in the implementation of referral guidelines for suspected haematological malignancies. The diagnosis is often made in the laboratory, and the clinical services become responsible for ensuring that the patient is seen within the time prescribed.[3] Patients with acute haematological malignancies may need to be seen within hours or days of diagnosis, whereas others with indolent disorders may require a long observation period before therapy is introduced. Close liaison with primary care is essential for best practice in all cases.

Secondary and tertiary care

Patients with haematological disorders require inpatient and outpatient facilities, high quality day care services, some instant access services, and increasing provision of care at home. The British Committee for Standards in Haematology (Clinical Task Force), a sub-committee of the British Society for Haematology, has recommended four levels of care, which reflect increasing diagnostic and therapeutic complexity.[4]

Level 1 offers high quality care for patients with general haematological disorders including a number of haematological malignancies. Among them are patients with slowly developing malignant diseases in a stable phase, and patients with malignant disease requiring chemotherapy that is unlikely to produce prolonged neutropenia, including multiple myeloma and myelodysplasias, managed using protocols that are not likely to produce marrow failure. The dual role of haematologists in the laboratory and clinical work requires that hospitals offering a Level 1 service should have a minimum of two consultant haematologists.

Level 2 aims to provide the services of Level 1 and also facilities for remission induction in acute myeloid or lymphoblastic leukaemia and lymphomas using intensive chemotherapy regimes. Level 2 care requires dedicated inpatient haematological teams with their own junior staff at SHO level and above, specially trained nurses and specially constructed facilities for the management of prolonged neutropenia. Such units should have a minimum of three consultant haematologists and ideally there should be collaboration between haematology and medical oncology if a medical oncology unit exists.

Level 3 care requires facilities for delivering autologous stem cell therapy associated with myeloablative chemotherapy regimes. Units offering Level 3 care require additional facilities for patient management, including stem cell harvesting and processing and high quality isolation facilities.

Level 4 care applies to units offering tertiary referral services, including allogeneic stem cell transplantation, specialist services in haemostasis and thrombosis and paediatric haematology services.

Although these gradings refer to the facilities needed for management of haematological malignancies, it is also appropriate to apply them to other specialised areas of haematological practice. Thus units at Levels 1, 2 and 3 may offer specialist services to cover one or more other aspects of haematology, for example haemoglobinopathy, lymphoma, acquired bleeding disorders or transfusion practice. Where such specialist care is offered, there should be additional appropriately skilled consultant input. It should be noted that the quality of haematological care is best where there is close collaboration and teamwork between consultant haematologists, each with a common core of shared knowledge as well as providing their individual specialty expertise.

iii Special patterns of referral

Urgent referral

Patients with spontaneous haemorrhage or the appearance of purpura, and patients with fever and pallor should have an urgent blood count performed. This may show the presence of a low platelet count, acute leukaemia, bone marrow failure etc, requiring immediate referral. Patients with suspected lymphoma, as evidenced by a persistent lymphadenopathy, often accompanied by night sweats and weight loss, should be referred to be seen within two weeks.[3] All hospitals should be able to provide a 24-hour consultant led cover for such emergencies from primary care, besides dealing with urgent requests from other hospital-based units to deal with problems of bleeding, haemostasis, or thrombosis. A major part of general haematology is the investigation and treatment of anaemia, referral often coming from secondary care.

Tertiary referral

Tertiary referrals are to centres with particular expertise and facilities. Such referral is most commonly for allogeneic haematopoietic stem cell transplantation, to centres with specialist skills in the management of haemostatic disorders or with experience in rare life-threatening haematological disorders. Patients with haemophilia are referred to centres that operate comprehensive services, including specialist orthopaedic and physiotherapy services. Tertiary referral may also occur at a regional level where special procedures are required within a comprehensive care plan. Many haematologists also provide a service in the interpretation of pathological specimens, including bone marrow and peripheral blood, morphology of lymph nodes, and immuno-phenotyping of lymphocytes and gene rearrangements thereof. In most tertiary centres offering specialist care there is a linked research programme.

iv Clinical networks and shared care

Many disorders of the blood are protracted. Some, such as inherited disorders, are lifelong. Some require prolonged intensive treatment, and others pursue a relapsing and remitting course or stable phase punctuated by acute emergencies. Such a catalogue of disorders lends itself to integrated care within a network system whereby the patient is managed jointly between primary care and the local hospital, with tertiary referral centres aware of the patients and their conditions and ready to give advice and help in an acute situation. For many years the very nature of these diseases has engendered a culture of networking amongst haematologists, though mainly this has been informal. The organisation of haemophilia services and the inclusive nature of the MRC Leukaemia Trials groups are good examples of such networking. More formal arrangements are being established, particularly in haemato-oncology. The majority of patients with haematological malignancies are in the older age group, and the greater the amount of informed care that can given locally, the better. Similar informal networks exist for the management of haemorrhagic disorders, particularly the inherited bleeding disorders and for families with thrombophilia. Particularly important networks or collaborations need to be in place for anticoagulant control. Whether this service is based mainly in the community or in the local hospital varies according to local arrangements, but scrupulous quality control and immediate access for patients with problems linked to the anticoagulation are essential.

v Requirements for a high quality service

The foundation for a high quality haematology service is the integration of clinical and laboratory expertise. As indicated above, as the degree of complexity of services offered increases so does the requirement for staff, facilities, training and skills. Levels 1–4 were introduced for haemato-oncology services[4] but the system can be applied to haematology in general.

Level 1

Level 1 is the provision of a safe, effective and helpful haematological service for primary care and the general working of the hospital. It includes the management of patients with haematological disorders requiring the expertise of the consultant but not the nursing or structural facilities needed to cope with prolonged neutropenia or other critical conditions. The main requirements are:

▪ A rapid results service for primary care, preferably through electronic links, coupled to ready access for interpretation of results and advice on management

▪ 24-hour service for other units within the hospital for advice on surgical, obstetrical or other general medical problems requiring haematological expertise

▪ participation in an active hospital transfusion committee, providing specialist advice on optimal transfusion requirements and safety

▪ a clear and dedicated system for anticoagulant control and

▪ treatment and management driven as far as possible by national evidence-based protocols.

Capital and staffing requirements

▪ A flexible number of specific haematology beds available on a general medical ward, the patients admitted under the care of the consultant haematologist

▪ bed services that include at least one room where neutropenic patients can be managed, protected from infection

▪ 24-hour consultant cover and 24-hour cover by doctors in training at SHO or SpR level, either dedicated to haematology or shared with the general medical team

▪ procedures that are protocol led

▪ nurses involved in the care of haematology patients should have at least six months' training in haematology or oncology and there should be access to the advice of a clinical nurse specialist

▮ services for intravenous administration of blood products, antibiotics and chemotherapy should be available throughout the 24 hours and

▮ ready access to medical microbiology services and pharmacists with particular expertise in chemotherapy.

Outpatient services

There should be dedicated outpatient clinics with appropriate support staff, with phlebotomy and laboratory services so that patients attending outpatients receive prompt advice and care based upon the results of the blood count where this is appropriate.

Day care

Much of the service, including transfusions and some chemotherapy, can be delivered through day care. This may be linked to a home delivery system. Day care units need a specialist nursing complement, though the facilities may be shared with other units. There must be consultant cover at all times.

Staffing

The minimum requirement is two consultant haematologists with dedicated or shared junior staff able to provide continuous 24-hour cover. As the population served increases, and if there are specialist surgical, obstetric or other specialist services requiring haematological input, so the need for a third consultant haematologist soon becomes apparent. Compliance with NHS directives on *A Better Blood Transfusion*[5] and *Referral Guidelines for Suspected Cancer*[3] means that most large district general hospitals at Level 1 require a third haematology consultant.

Level 2

The staffing and capital requirements are as for Level 1 but with certain additions.

▮ Haematology beds need to be grouped together, with access to isolation facilities where standard chemotherapy protocols may be administered and patients managed safely through prolonged periods of neutropenia

▮ Haematological cover must be available at all times, and there should be dedicated staff in training

▮ There must be 24-hour microbiological cover and centralised pharmacy facilities for makeup of chemotherapy, and appropriate imaging techniques.

Level 2 facilities require a minimum of three haematologists to provide the full range of expertise and cover.

Level 3

The additional requirements above Level 2 are for increased expertise from medical, nursing and pharmacy staff for intravenous therapies, including central venous lines, as well as the cytopheresis facilities for stem cell collection. If the Level 3 is for haemato-oncology there needs to be multidisciplinary working with medical microbiology, histopathology, pathology and imaging departments. If other specialist haematological services are offered, the appropriate skills and equipment will need to be in place.

Level 4

- Full isolation facilities for stem cell transplantation are required, with a dedicated transplant unit

- Appropriately trained nurses, pharmacists, physiotherapists and counsellors are required.

- Data management becomes an important part of the care of patients, and a data manager is essential (much of the work at Levels 3 and 4 being protocol driven or done within national or international clinical trials, and reports to the appropriate data registries are mandatory for audit and clinical governance)

- Other specialist services, particularly in the realm of thrombophilia and haemostasis, may be offered and appropriately trained staff and facilities are required

- Where transplantation is offered units should have a minimum of two consultants with experience in stem cell transplantation as well as the appropriate complement of consultant haematologists to cover hospital requirements

- Training for specialist SpRs, undergraduate teaching and postgraduate courses, clinical governance and with enough time to maintain continuing professional development

- The nursing and capital facilities required have been laid down by a number of guidelines conforming to European standards and include dedicated transplant isolation rooms with filtered air, a particular nursing complement, pharmacy conforming to chemotherapy guidelines and stem cell collection facilities which meet strict criteria.

Most Level 4 units are in teaching hospitals where other specialist units require an increased input from haematologists. Such units require at least five consultants to cover service work plus the additional complement for academic medicine.

vi   Clinical work of consultants in haematology

It will be appreciated that there is a considerable variation in the type of work carried out by individual consultant haematologists, depending upon their specialisation and clinical practice. Most consultants have two or three timetabled outpatient sessions a week, often with some degree of specialisation in one or more of the clinics. Outpatient time may be shared between two or more consultants, or the total number of clinics for the unit extended. Formal ward rounds should take place twice a week with a multidisciplinary team that includes junior staff, nursing specialists and pharmacists, with input from dietitians and social workers. For care at Levels 2 and 3, daily chart rounds by a consultant haematologist are advisable, and they are mandatory at Level 4. A major part of the consultant haematologist's duty is to review the daily laboratory results from the various units, diagnostic, haemostasis and thrombosis, transfusion and so on, and interface with the other units in the hospital and primary care. In addition to clinical work, the consultant haematologist has overall responsibility for the quality assurance schemes of the haematology laboratory. A consultant haematologist also has responsibility for day care units and needs to be available for consultation if required by the nursing staff or training grade doctors. Combined clinics may be required with other specialties for example, clinical oncologists and possibly surgeons in joint lymphoma clinics, with orthopaedic surgeons and other specialists in haemophilia clinics; and the maintenance of an anti-coagulant service and with paediatricians where there is no separate paediatric haematology service.

vii Multidisciplinary team working

Multidisciplinary working is essential to good practice in haematology, the requirements increasing with the level of care. Nurse practitioners practise widely in haematology. They may have special expertise in transfusion medicine, haemato-oncology, haemostasis and thrombosis, haemophilia, anticoagulant services and apheresis services. Levels 3 and 4 care require dedicated medical microbiologists with a special interest in haematological problems, particularly those of immunosuppressed and neutropenic patients. Close collaboration with imaging services and pathology is essential for diagnosis and management. Special pharmacy services for chemotherapy and antibiotic management are an essential part of haemato-oncology. At the higher levels a dedicated dietitian is helpful. At Levels 3 and 4, there must be close liaison with ward cleaning services and the infection control team.

viii Conjoined services

Services conjoined to a haematology service are:

- nursing – specialist haematology nurses, IV teams, haemophilia nurses, anticoagulant nurses
- medical microbiology, infection disease control
- specialised histopathology services
- community care services for haemoglobinopathies and haemophilia
- imaging services
- data management
- patient and family counselling services
- patient support groups and appropriate charities.

ix Specialised facilities required

Some indication of the specialised facilities required has been given above. These depend to some extent on the nature of the specialised services offered.

Outpatients

Outpatient facilities need to be appropriate for the type of service offered. Many haematological disorders are serious, indeed life-threatening, and proper facilities, with privacy for counselling and breaking of bad news, need to be available in the outpatient department. Outpatients should also be reasonably close to the haematology laboratory.

Day care facilities

These should contain appropriate chairs or beds at stations for transfusion regimes, outpatient chemotherapy and rapid access service. Haemophilia patients require their own rapid access points.

There must be a separate area for therapeutic apheresis and cytopheresis. Such services are normally offered where stem cell collection is provided. This should have a dedicated area, and the processing of stem cells must meet national and European standards. Facilities for insertion of central lines and a full range of intravenous pumps and drug delivery systems must be available to the day care and inpatient staff. Adequate day care space and equipment reduces the need for inpatient accommodation.

Inpatients

Most haematology units require isolation rooms for the management of immunosuppressed or neutropenic patients, together with expertise in intravenous lines and pumps. At Levels 3 and 4 there must be equipment for monitoring cardiac and pulmonary function, haemoglobin saturation and other vital signs, and a specially constructed space with filtered air and positive pressure rooms. For severely immunosuppressed and transplant patients such spaces need an anteroom for scrub-up and they must be large enough to accept imaging machinery for patients who cannot leave their room.

x Quality standards

▯ *National and international trials.* Where possible, patients with acute leukaemia, lymphoma and myeloma should be managed within the protocols of national or international trials, with reports made to those studies. Audit is then relatively straightforward in relation to outcome in any unit, or at least the standards that are to be achieved are known.

▯ *National guidelines.* Most procedures in haematology are now governed by national guidelines, which should be familiar throughout the unit.

▯ *Cancer and transplant registries.* Where appropriate, patients should be reported to cancer registries or to the international or European bone marrow transplant registries. Safety and quality are best assured through protocol-driven therapy and participation in local, regional and national audit programmes. This applies not only to haemato-oncology but also to haemophilia, anticoagulant control services and specialist services offered for uncommon disorders both inherited and acquired.

▯ *Laboratory standards* are assured through National External Quality Assurance Schemes and Clinical Pathology Accreditation (CPA).

xi Contribution to acute medicine

Haematologists are rarely directly involved in the delivery of care in general internal medicine but contribute hugely through specialist knowledge to the management of patients in acute medicine. Contact and collaboration often arise through the laboratory route, whence come the generalist skills of the haematologist.

xii Academic haematology

Haematology has a high proportion of consultants with academic qualifications. Most Level 4 units and many others have major academic departments. The NHS duties of the academic staff are best channelled towards the clinical side of their research interests. Academic haematologists usually take their share of on-call commitments and offer scheduled outpatient, day care, and inpatient services for management of patients with specialist problems.

xiii Developments to improve patient care

Therapeutics

- New drugs, particularly biological products engineered to target specific malignant cell types, are very expensive but offer the prospect of better control of haematological malignancies.

- Recombinant coagulation factors, not only Factor VIII and Factor IX but many other factors, offer the prospect of safe and more effective control of a number of disorders. Among them are inherited disorders such as haemophilia and other coagulation deficiencies, and acquired disorders, including acute sepsis and diffuse intravascular coagulation, massive haemorrhage, and surgical blood loss.

- An extending range of antibiotics is proving of great benefit in the management of immunosuppressed and neutropenic patients.

- Lipid formulations of some drugs, which otherwise have specific organ toxicity, offer improved prospects for chemotherapy and antimicrobial therapies.

Community care and therapy

- Improved drug delivery systems linked to intravenous or subcutaneous access will allow more patients to be managed at home or as day cases.

- Devices which offer the option of home or primary care control of anticoagulant therapy should improve the quality of life of ambulatory and otherwise normal patients.

Stem cell transplantation

Advances in stem cell transplantation, including non-ablative conditioning regimens and immune modulation, may extend the indications for stem cell transplantation and reduce transplant-related mortality.

Nurse practitioners

Nurse practitioners with specialist training and skills have been introduced to many branches of haematology and this aspect of care needs to be expanded. Nurse-led teams for the insertion of central lines, haemophilia nurses, nurse counsellors for haemoglobinopathies, transfusion nurses and nurses to lead intravenous teams are in place in some units. More of them will greatly aid patient care. In many instances liaison with community nursing produces great benefits.

WORK OF CONSULTANTS IN HAEMATOLOGY

1 Direct patient care

A Work in the specialty

Inpatient work

- Ward rounds with specialist nurses, pharmacists and other members of the healthcare team. There should be a minimum of two per week; and there should be daily chart rounds with nursing and training grade staff in specialist units. Teaching and training are important components of the main ward rounds.

- Referral for haematological advice, particularly in transfusion, haemostasis and thrombosis and anticoagulant control, and for diagnosis in patients with fever of undiagnosed origin, are common in most hospitals. Such referrals usually require close liaison with laboratory staff besides clinical skills.

- Patients with acute haematological malignancies may often present directly to inpatients rather than via outpatient clinics.

The inpatient load of a full time consultant should be no more than 250 inpatients, this figure applying mainly to care at Levels 1 and 2. This figure must be reduced to allow for the additional time required for management of acute episodes in haemato-oncology.

Outpatient clinics

The annual clinical activity per consultant recommended is 250 new patients and 1,500 follow-up, plus 1,500 day case/ward attendees.[7] This would suggest six new haematology patients per week, with up to 10 follow-up cases per clinic, though again there is considerable variation according to the nature of the haematology practice and the complexity of the cases. Time has to be available for proper explanation and counselling of patients who have been found to have malignant diseases, particularly leukaemias and lymphomas and other life-threatening conditions.

Subspecialty clinics within haematology

- Thrombophilia clinics – including genetic counselling
- Joint lymphoma clinics
- Haemoglobinopathy clinics with counselling/antenatal screening and advice
- Haemato-oncology follow-up including chemotherapy
- Anticoagulant and thrombosis services
- Paediatric services with appropriately trained paediatric staff
- National Blood Transfusion Services.

B Acute medicine

Haematologists are rarely directly involved in the delivery of care in general internal medicine (but see xi above).

C Academic medicine

Haematologists with academic contracts should not expect to devote more than six sessions to NHS service work if their academic work is to flourish. Ideally clinical and academic activities should be complementary.

2 Work to maintain and improve the quality of care

This work encompasses duties in clinical governance, professional self-regulation, continuing professional development, education and training of others. For many consultants, at various times in their careers, it may include research, serving in management, and providing advice. All require consultant participation. Such work is described fully in Part 1 of this document. Its scope is summarised in the Appendix to Part 2. Management and advisory work are identified specifically in the Appendix.

WORKFORCE REQUIREMENTS FOR HAEMATOLOGY

A number of initiatives have put additional requirements on the work of haematologists, including *Better blood transfusion*[5] and the *NHS cancer plan.*[6] The British Society of Haematology and the Joint Intercollegiate Committee of Haematology, involving the Royal Colleges of Physicians and the Royal College of Pathologists, together with the Specialist Workforce Advisory Group, estimate that an extra 250 haematologists will be required in England over the next seven years.[7] At least 149 of these are needed to implement the NHS Cancer Plan. The numbers do not include expansion in paediatric haematology or transfusion medicine.

There should be at least two consultant haematologists in an acute trust offering laboratory and clinical services. Most acute DGHs should have three and those serving a population >450,000 need four.[8] Units offering Level 4 services and academic units require a minimum of five consultants.

The present workforce averages 1.4 consultants per trust, 2.1 per acute DGH. There is wide variation across the country in the distribution that makes up the average, and the number per acute DGH is elevated by the inclusion of teaching hospital units. When calculating the number of consultant haematologists required, it is important to include the work on the laboratory side. The Clinical Bench Marking Company[9] has shown that in haematology the median excess of sessions (notional half-days) across the UK is 6.5. The total NHD worked is from 16 to 26, grossly in excess of recommended workload.[10]

It can be seen from the figures of the current workload that there is a considerable under-provision of consultant haematologists to provide a comprehensive, safe and prompt service that patients and their families expect. This document has set out a working framework for consultant haematologists, indicating that the number of consultants per acute district general hospital should be over three, based upon general and special haematology duties. Calculations based on the annual number of laboratory requests also indicate that there is a >50% shortfall in consultant numbers to support the expanding specialist units as well as acute surgery and medicine of a similar proportion.[9] Pressures are driven in part by the increasing expectations of the population, but in particular by the NHS Cancer Plan[11], the two-week wait, the drive for better blood transfusion practice, as well as the practical success of more complex and intensive therapeutic regimens.

In addition to the drive for higher quality clinical care, there are the requirements to measure and maintain that quality through clinical governance and continuing professional development.[11] In clinical haematology this means, in part, participation in national or international clinical trials. In many cases patients are not entered into appropriate studies because of the time requirements for proper documentation and audit. Time for such work needs to be included in any job plans for a consultant haematologist, together with time for updating knowledge and skills.

The proposed expansion of 50% in consultant numbers, with appropriate expansion of SpR posts, will still leave a shortfall in the optimal number of consultant haematologists. The expansion of consultant numbers from 1996 to 1998 was <1% with an 8% expansion in 1999. An expansion of 10% per annum at least would be appropriate for providing a high quality service and the urgent need at this stage is to expand the training grade to cater to this need.

It should be noted that this review of workforce requirements does not take into account expanding needs in paediatric haematology nor in transfusion services. Consultant numbers in these specialties are currently included in the overall haematology consultant count.

References

1. Cartwright RA, Gilman EA, Gurney KA. The trends in incidence of haematological and related conditions. *Br J Haematol* 106:281–295;(1999).

2. Cartwright RA, Brinker H, Carli PM, *et al.* The rise in incidence in lymphoma in Europe 1985–1992. *Eur J Cancer* 1999;**35**:627–633.

3. *Referral guidelines for suspected cancer.* NHS Executive (April, 2000).

4. British Committee for Standards in Haematology. Guidelines on the provision of facilities for the care of adult patients with haematological malignancies. *Clin Lab Haematol* 1995;**17**:1–10.

5. *Better blood transfusion.* Health Service Circular HSC1998/224 (December,1998).

6. *The NHS Cancer Plan. A plan for investment. A plan for reform.* NHS (September 2000).

7. *Haematology Consultant Manpower in the Twenty-first Century.* A Joint Intercollegiate Committee on Haematology/ British Society for Haematology Document (January 2001).

8. Haematology Consultant Manpower in the Twenty-first Century. A Joint Intercollegiate Committee on Haematology/British Society for Haematology Document (January 2001).

9. Clinical Benchmarking Company Ltd. Annual Reports (1996/7; 1997/8; 1998/9).

10. Royal College of Physicians. *Consultant physicians working for patients.* London: RCP, 1999.

11. Department of Health. *A first class service; quality in the new NHS.* London: DoH, 1998.

Immunology

i   Introduction: a brief description of the specialty and clinical needs of patients

The clinical practice of immunology, as defined by the World Health Organisation (WHO), encompasses clinical and laboratory activity dealing with the study, diagnosis and management of patients with diseases resulting from disordered immunological mechanisms, and conditions in which immunological manipulations form an important part of therapy.[1] In the UK, the practice of immunology largely conforms to this WHO definition, with immunologists providing combined clinical and laboratory services for patients with immunodeficiency, autoimmune disease, systemic vasculitis and allergy.

Allergy has recently been recognised as a specialty in its own right. Historically, however, in view of the immunological principles underlying allergic disease and the patchy development of allergy services, many immunologists have set up and continue to provide a significant allergy service including desensitisation therapy, as there are insufficient specialist allergists in the NHS at present.

ii   Organisation of the service

Clinical immunology has evolved over the past two decades from a laboratory base to a combined clinical and laboratory specialty. A typical immunology service is based in a teaching hospital and led by a consultant immunologist, and comprises a mixture of clinical and laboratory staff. The clinical team will include specialist registrars in immunology and immunology nurse specialists, while the laboratory team is comprised of bio-medical and clinical scientists.

The advent of laboratory accreditation has led many district general hospitals to seek formal consultant immunology input into their diagnostic immunology services. In many instances laboratory duties are combined with clinical work.

The catchment area of the service not only includes the immediate population served by the Trust but often extends to the population of the wider region.

iii   Ways of working

Immunologists work as members of multidisciplinary teams that include nurse specialists. Nurse specialists in immunology play a leading role in all aspects of immunoglobulin infusion, ranging from supervision of hospital clinics to the training and supervision of patients who undertake self-infusion of immunoglobulin as part of the home therapy programme. In many centres, immunology nurse specialists also undertake skin testing for allergy and provide training on the use of self-injectable adrenaline for patients with life-threatening allergic disease.

Several other complementary services are essential for the efficient delivery of a good immunology service. A comprehensive diagnostic immunology laboratory underpins the diagnosis of all immunological disease.

In view of the propensity of antibody deficient patients to develop complications involving multiple organ systems, there must be close liaison with colleagues in a range of specialties including respiratory medicine, ENT surgery, haematology, ophthalmology and gastroenterology. Access to specialist microbiology and virology laboratories is vital for the early detection and optimal management of the infectious complications of immunodeficiency.

iv Outline of clinical and laboratory work in the specialty

Direct patient care

The clinical work of consultant immunologists is largely out-patient based, with the following broad work patterns.

▮ Immunologists are solely responsible for patients with primary immunodeficiency (antibody deficiency, combined T and B cell deficiency, complement deficiency and phagocytic defects).

▮ In centres without dedicated allergists, patients with severe allergic disease (food allergy, drug allergy, venom allergy, anaphylaxis) are also looked after primarily by consultant immunologists.

▮ In most centres consultant immunologists perform joint clinics with paediatricians to cater for children with immunodeficiency and allergy.

▮ Many immunologists have an interest in connective tissue disease and perform joint clinics with rheumatologists for patients with autoimmune rheumatic disease and systemic vasculitis.

▮ Immunoglobulin infusion clinics for patients with antibody deficiency form an integral part of the clinical workload of consultant immunologists. A recent audit of primary antibody deficiency in the UK and discussions within the specialty, suggest that a single consultant should be responsible for a maximum of 50 patients with antibody deficiency in order to deliver optimum care.[2] With the increasing recognition of intravenous immunoglobulin as a therapeutic immuno-modulator, these infusion clinics have expanded in some centres to include non-antibody deficient patients, eg inflammatory neuropathies.

Junior medical staff support

Outpatient clinics are run in many centres with the help of specialist registrars in immunology. Since many SpRs have had little or no previous experience in immunology, consultant supervision of training is essential. The time required for supervision will thus limit the number of patients who can be seen by a consultant.

Laboratory immunology

Consultant immunologists are responsible for directing diagnostic immunology services and perform a wide range of duties including clinical liaison, interpretation and validation of results, quality assurance, assay development and supervision of bio-medical and clinical scientists and specialist registrars. Some consultants perform a limited amount of 'hands on' laboratory work.

In view of the work pressures on immunologists, it is felt that consultants undertaking supervision of laboratories outwith their base hospital should devote not more than one session a week for such duties, and should therefore be associated with only one additional hospital.

v   Quality of service

The quality of the laboratory immunology service has been underpinned since 1993 by accreditation by Clinical Pathology Accreditation (UK Ltd) and plans for accreditation of clinical services in respect of immunodeficiency are actively underway as part of the UK Primary Immunodeficiency Network.

WORK OF CONSULTANTS IN IMMUNOLOGY

1   Direct patient care

A Work in the specialty

Outpatient work, including day cases

▪ Primary immunodeficiency clinics

▪ Severe allergic disease clinics

> The complexity of clinical referrals requires that sufficient time is spent on assessing patients at the first consultation which necessarily limits the number of patients who can be seen in a single outpatient session. A consultant immunologist working alone will typically see 5–10 patients (new and old) in a session of one NHD, depending to the complexity of the problem.

▪ Joint clinics with paediatricians for children with immunodeficiency and allergy

▪ Joint clinics with rheumatologists

▪ Immunoglobulin infusion clinics

▪ A consultant should be responsible for a maximum of 50 patients with antibody deficiency in order to deliver optimum care.[2]

Inpatient work

Inpatient referrals (see section iii above)

Overall it is envisaged that a consultant immunologist will require 4–5 NHDs for clinical activity in out-patients, day case units and to see ward referrals.

Laboratory work (see sections iii, iv above)

In general a consultant immunologist will require 4–5 NHDs to fulfil these responsibilities.

B Acute medicine

Immunologists do not participate in the on-take rota for unselected medical emergencies.

C Academic medicine

The NHS workload of academic clinical immunologists depends on their academic responsibilities and individual job descriptions, but in general they make a strong contribution to the work of the NHS department.

2. Work to maintain and improve the quality of care

This work encompasses duties in clinical governance, professional self-regulation, continuing professional development, education and training of others. For many consultants, at various times in their careers, it may include research, serving in management, and providing advice. All require consultant participation. Such work is described fully in Part 1 of this document. Its scope is summarised in the Appendix to Part 2. Management and advisory work are identified specifically in the Appendix.

WORKFORCE REQUIREMENTS FOR IMMUNOLOGY

There are only limited data available on the workload of immunologists, who are based mainly in teaching hospitals. Increasing awareness of immunological diseases, coupled with the need to provide specialist advice and direction to immunology laboratories, including those in larger district general hospitals, has placed a traditionally understaffed specialty with many single-handed consultants under great strain.

An estimate of the number of consultant immunologists required in England and Wales is based upon the recent workload survey undertaken by the Royal College of Pathologists[3] and extensive consultation within the specialty. The survey showed that consultant immunologists currently work a median of 57 hours a week (16.3 NHDs) performing the various activities detailed above. Workforce requirements have been calculated on the basis that:

- most immunologists are based in teaching hospitals
- the population served by existing consultant immunologists is 38.9 million.

Assuming that each consultant will not be expected to exceed his or her contractual obligation of 11 NHDs, it is estimated that 97 whole time consultants in immunology are required to serve the total population of England and Wales (53.4 million). This translates into 1 consultant immunologist per 550,000 of the population compared to the existing provision of 1 per 1.1 million of the population. The current consultant establishment of 49 immunologists falls short of this figure by 48. Consultant expansion of 4.7% per annum will therefore be required over the next 10 years to achieve this figure.

NOTE: *In 1999 there was insufficient information available to allow a more precise estimate of the workforce requirements in this specialty. This recent estimate provides a firmer basis for workforce planning but this too will need to be reviewed in the light of developments in practice and service delivery.*

Annex: Example of the work programme of a consultant immunologist

Activity	Workload	NHDs
Direct patient care		
Out-patient clinics	5–10 patients per clinic	3–4
New patients	3–4 patients per clinic	
Follow-up patients	6–8 patients per clinic	
IV Ig infusion	6–10 patients per clinic	
Ward consultation and telephone advice		0.5
Allergy, including desensitisation immunotherapy		1
Total direct patient care		*4–5*
Laboratory work		
Clinical liaison, interpretation of results		
Quality assurance		
Supervision of trainees		
Assay development		
'Hands on' laboratory work		
Supervision of district general hospital immunology laboratories		
Total laboratory work		*4–5*
Work to maintain and improve the quality of care		**2–4**

References

1. Lambert *et al*. Clinical Immunology: guidelines for its organisation, training and certification: relationships with allergology and other medical disciplines – a WHO/IUIS/IAACI report. *Clinical and Experimental Immunology* 1993;**93**:484–91.

2. Spickett GP, Ashew T, Chapel HM. Development of primary antibody deficiency by consultant immunologists in the UK: a paradigm for other rare diseases. *Quality in Health Care* 1995;**4**:263–8.

3. Medical and Scientific Staffing of the National Health Service Pathology Departments. Royal College of Pathologists June 1999.

Infectious diseases (including tropical medicine)

i Introduction: a brief description of the specialty and the clinical needs of patients

Background

Historically, infectious diseases was one of the earliest medical subspecialties. Communicable diseases units (as they were then called) were established, usually based on fever hospitals, which were located in the depths of the countryside for fear of spreading pestilence to the community. They served as centres of expertise for diseases such as hepatitis, meningitis, infective diarrhoea, measles, polio, diphtheria and smallpox.

During the 1950s and 1960s there was a widespread belief that infectious diseases were largely overcome, at least in the developed world. Improvements in public health, new vaccines and the availability of antibiotics together had a profound effect on the "classical" infectious diseases. As a result, many of the fever hospitals were closed and the number of specialists in infectious diseases declined to near extinction.

This optimism was short-lived. By the late 1970s and early 1980s it became clear that infection was re-emerging as a major source of public health concern. 'New' infections such as Legionnaire's disease, toxic shock syndrome, helicobacter and campylobacter infections and of course, HIV, all conspired to put infection 'back on the map'. As modern medical and surgical management have become more complex there are more immunosuppressed patients in hospitals vulnerable to infection. More recently there has been major emphasis at the highest level on containment and control of hospital-acquired infections, appropriate use of antibiotics and control of antibiotic resistance and the growing public interest in food hygiene related illnesses.[1,2]

Simultaneously, there was a re-emerging interest in infection as an academic specialty and as a result, during the last 15 years, infectious diseases has grown rapidly, although from an extremely small base. The pattern now is increasingly for academic units in infectious diseases to be established within major multi-disciplinary medical centres.

The present

The specialty of clinical infectious disease (ID) is an internationally recognised specialty. It offers clinical care for patients who have a communicable condition that can spread from human to human, whom therefore it might be necessary to manage in an isolation facility. Examples might include viral haemorrhagic fever, multi-drug resistant tuberculosis, MRSA and salmonella gastroenteritis. It also provides specialist knowledge and expertise that might be needed for diagnosis and management in, for example fever of uncertain origin, unexplained jaundice in a returning traveller, the assessment of a petechial rash, chronic fatigue syndrome, and rigors or injecting drug user. ID physicians are also trained to look after patients with HIV/AIDS and/or viral hepatitis. In addition, because of the shortage of tropical physicians in the UK (see below) they usually offer specialist clinical services for ill returning travellers (including tourists and travellers for commercial, military or healthcare purposes) or visitors to the UK (including tourists and refugees). ID is one of the few medical specialties in which new diseases and new organisms regularly emerge. ID physicians must therefore remain informed about wider developments in their specialty, as well as diagnostic and therapeutic developments, if they are to fulfill the infection needs of the community and institutions they serve.[3,4]

There is considerable overlap in the function of ID specialists and clinical microbiologists in providing advice on the diagnosis and management of patients with potential infective problems and in advising Trusts on infection control, formulary and similar issues. Where the services co-exist in a hospital a combined consultation team has been shown to be effective[5,6] and there is some published evidence for the additional benefit of ID advice as well as that provided by microbiologists.[7,8] In some countries it is normal for specialist training in ID to include substantive training in microbiology. This model is now being trialled in a small number of centres in the UK.[9,10]

Some consultant level specialists in tropical medicine practice in association with a few English teaching hospitals, and they normally function as academic physicians. Training in tropical medicine is an extension of ID training, with additional emphasis upon time spent training in a tropical country and the undertaking of specialist courses of instruction and appropriate qualifications such as the courses leading to the Diploma in Tropical Medicine and Hygiene (DTM&H) and/or a Masters degree in Tropical Medicine.[11] Specialists in tropical medicine will usually possess a high level of advanced knowledge in their field, and this specialised knowledge may be accessed by consultants in ID and other specialities working in other parts of the UK and beyond.

ii   Organisation of ID services at primary, secondary and tertiary levels

Most tertiary British specialist ID services are based in teaching hospitals or in large district general hospitals (DGHs). In such centres there should be at least two WTE consultants (usually more) in ID. Each consultant is typically responsible for 500 finished consultant episodes (FCEs) and 750–1000 outpatient visits per year (excluding travel medicine clinics). Fifty per cent of ID physicians also have a formal commitment to general internal medicine and a high proportion of patients referred to specialist ID units turn out to have a non-infectious diagnosis.[12,13] Similar regional ID services specifically targeted at children also exist in some teaching centres. All ID physicians work closely with local public health services and laboratory-based microbiology services to assist with the control of communicable disease in the population at large. Some large centres in the UK, including some teaching hospitals, do not have an ID unit with beds staffed by CCST-holding ID physicians. In these and in most DGHs, the first point of call for infection advice is the clinical microbiologist. Recent reports have repeated earlier joint Colleges recommendations that such hospitals should also have an ID physician specialist to complement such advice.[14,15,16]

iii   Special patterns of referral

These vary locally but often include referrals from general practitioners, from consultants in other specialities within teaching hospitals, from consultants in district general hospitals, referrals that are part of an established consultation service (eg bacteraemia service), patient self-referral (eg travel clinics, HIV/AIDS services), and referrals from drug addiction services (eg HIV/AIDS cases, viral hepatitis cases) etc.

iv Ways of working in ID, with reference to clinical networks and community arrangements

Specialists in ID will provide inpatient and outpatient opinions. Some ID physicians run services located in places outside the hospital, depending upon local clinical needs (eg prison clinics for hepatitis C and HIV/AIDS). To do this effectively, ID physicians will ensure that hospital-based medical colleagues, laboratory colleagues, general practitioners and public health services are made aware of the ID services available locally. Because of the relative scarcity of specialised expertise in many aspects of ID and tropical medicine, information and advice is often sought from ID and tropical physicians via telephone and e-mail by colleagues in general practice, in hospital medicine, in public health, and in paramedical services (eg travel medicine nurses, drug addiction services). This aspect of daily workload is difficult to quantify but needs due recognition in work plans.

v Characteristics of a high quality service, and the requirements for ensuring this

To practise high-quality ID it is essential that there is a well-functioning team. Some members may be attached more loosely than others but an excellent team spirit valuing the contribution of all is of the greatest value. The team would ideally include medical CCST-holding consultants and dedicated medical trainees. There should be a strong educational and research ethos in a constantly changing specialty which often has a high public profile. Nursing staff must be familiar with communicable diseases work, including minimisation of cross infection, and be able to work with 'high-risk' patients. Where appropriate the team should include community nurses, health visitors and professions allied to medicine. The last include physiotherapists, occupational therapists, speech therapists, psychologists, non-medical specialists in addiction (for drug use-related problems), pharmacists (because of complex polypharmacy), dietitians, social workers and counsellors.

vi The clinical work of consultants in the specialty

Consultants are responsible for providing clinical leadership, providing clinical services (with the assistance of their junior staff) and creating and developing new and improved services for patients based upon local needs. Consultants also have teaching and training duties (medical students, junior doctors, peers, nurses, PAMS etc) both in the NHS and in association with local medical schools, and they will have a commitment to research. They also have wider advisory and administrative roles.

vii The work of the other members of the multidisciplinary team

Junior doctors work under the direction of consultants to provide high quality services for patients. Nurses create a high quality safe environment for investigation and management, with minimal risk both to patients and to the public at large. PAMS ensure that the patient is looked after holistically by working diligently within their personal field of expertise. Like doctors, nurses and PAMS should not only be involved in patient care but should also be involved in teaching, training and have a commitment to research devoted towards helping patients.

viii Conjoined care

ID Physicians collaborate with microbiologists, virologists, public health physicians, psychiatrists specialising in drug addiction, and ITU specialists (for life-threatening infections). Where PAMS are not closely managerially integrated into the ID team close working arrangements should be fostered. Depending on patient and community needs, ID services may also collaborate with other services, such as general practice, terminal care, hepatology/gastroenterology services (for viral hepatitis and advanced liver disease), respiratory medicine (for tuberculosis), genitourinary medicine (eg for HIV/AIDS), obstetric services and paediatric services (eg for perinatal and family management of HIV, viral hepatitis), long-term residential care facilities, community-based voluntary services, travel health services, immunology services, and specialist tropical medicine services

ix Specialised facilities required

ID physicians require access to single rooms offering positive and negative pressure isolation facilities. The former is necessary for the management of patients with severe immunosuppression problems, the latter for patients infected with hazardous organisms such as chickenpox and multi-drug resistant tuberculosis. Because of the nature of the pathologies some ID patients can be very ill (eg meningococcal septicaemia, falciparum malaria, toxic shock syndrome, Legionnaire's Disease) and close access to expert resuscitation support and to intensive care facilities is necessary. Additional specialist equipment, such as access to a Trexler isolator unit is only rarely needed (eg for a possible case of Lassa Fever), but possession of facilities for accommodating such patients safely, and access to the means for transporting them to an appropriate unit are essential.

x Quality standards and measures of the quality of the specialised service

Staff in ID services should engage in regular internal and external teaching and training, including peer education for consultants. Referral mechanisms and patterns should be under constant review to optimise service delivery. Risk management programmes and complaints review programmes should be in place to assess risk (real and perceived) and to address actual and potential problems and institute remedy. A programme of regular clinical and medical audit should be conducted. The British Infection Society has piloted a peer review scheme for external quality assurance of the functioning of specialist ID services/units, similar to schemes developed for example by the British Thoracic Society.

xi The contribution made by consultants in the specialty to acute medicine

ID contributes to acute medicine in many ways. ID units admit and look after acutely ill patients, both from the community and from other parts of the hospital. ID Consultants will advise on patients under the care of other hospital specialists, either through solicited or, depending upon local arrangements, unsolicited consultations. 50% of ID consultants also have general medical admitting duties;

xii **The duties, responsibilities and areas of work of academic physicians, with reference to NHS work**

A high proportion (55%) of English ID specialists and 80% of tropical medicine specialists hold contracts of employment with a university. They are based managerially within a medical school and have a number of clinical sessions devoted to work on the ID unit located in the adjacent teaching hospital (usually 6 out of 11 weekly sessions). Within the time limitations imposed by their academic duties, such ID academics carry part of the ID clinical workload, conduct clinical research and audit in the NHS setting, contribute politically and administratively to the NHS, and are involved in education and training of NHS staff and medical students intending careers in the NHS. Both the NHS and the universities should recognise and support this duality of role for academic ID physicians. In the case of the UK's tropical physicians, who usually hold academic contracts, their duties will be similar but their activity will be devoted towards tropical medicine issues.

xiii **Developments that offer improved patient care, and the conditions for introducing them into services**

Where there is adequate team staffing, specialist clinics dealing with TB, HIV/AIDS, viral hepatitis, travel medicine, immunisation, returning travellers, and chronic fatigue syndrome represent rewarding areas of expanded activity. Domiciliary antibiotic services, soft tissue sepsis services, and medical services for groups such as refugees, drug abusers, homeless people and travelling people are other expanded services that work (or have worked) successfully in some parts of the UK. Tropical physicians may develop tests, interpretative skills and services that will be of great value in the management of very difficult or unusual cases of imported disease (eg leprosy).

WORK OF CONSULTANTS IN INFECTIOUS DISEASES AND TROPICAL MEDICINE

1 Direct Patient Care

On-take and mandatory post-take rounds

On-call cover for most ID units is constant (24 hours per day, seven days per week) with a rota involving all ID consultant staff. Consultants are regularly on call overnight and over weekends regularly (1:2, 1:3 or 1:4). Post-take ward rounds are built into the general ward round activity of the ID unit. Consultants lead the round, or allow a specialist registrar to take the round and report subsequently.

Some geographically adjacent ID Units have cross-cover arrangements between their consultant staff to ensure adequate time for rest and other activities.

Consultants with general medical duties appear on the hospital's on-call rota with consultant physicians from other specialties. This should be no more often than for consultants in any other specialty. Given that ID consultants are often on call for their specialist unit, some adjustment of the general medical on-call commitment may be justified to maintain an equitable load across the consultant workforce.

Academics in ID are usually contractually limited to a portion of the week (often 6 out of 11 sessions), and the weekly clinical commitment should be reduced in proportion (approximately

55% of the full time physician's workload). However, it is likely to be a feature of specialist revalidation that all working physicians, including academics, must continue to function actively and regularly as working physicians in their specialty if they are to be able to continue to work as specialist physicians. Both the University and the NHS should recognise that academic ID physicians need to continue to work regularly in the practice of their specialty and yet cannot deliver a full 11/11 service every week.

Academics in some ID units may choose to construct their clinical commitment in other ways; eg full time on call for a period of months, and complete cessation of clinical duties for a period of months, equating overall to the equivalent of a weekly 6/11 sessional commitment over a year. The situation would be similar for tropical medicine physicians, although they will be expected to develop interests and services more relevant to tropical medicine within their allocated NHS time. Academic specialists in tropical medicine who spend most of their time overseas will need to ensure adequate clinical experience and practice within the UK or appropriate similar medical service to maintain clinical standards required for specialist practice in the UK.

Inpatient work

- *Ward rounds* Consultant-led supervisory and educational ward rounds on the Specialist Unit, in the company of trainee junior doctors.
- *Referral work* Seeing and assessing solicited (and possibly) unsolicited consultations, dependent on local arrangements. Initial opinion may be by the consultant or by the specialist registrar with subsequent consultant review.
- *Inter-specialty and inter-disciplinary liaison* Include hospital grand rounds, internal departmental clinical meetings, clinico-pathological conferences, clinico-radiological conferences, attendance at the clinical meetings of other units where mutual patients are being discussed.
- *Case conferences* Multidisciplinary team work, looking at patient areas such as the HIV/AIDS patients, viral hepatitis patients, TB patients.

Academic ID consultants will have such duties, but these should be scaled down in line with the level of their clinical commitment. Consultants with a commitment to general internal medicine are likely to have equivalent duties and on-call commitments on other wards, including dedicated post-take rounds, besides their specialty work.

Outpatient clinics

- *Specialty clinics* One to three clinics per week.
- *New patients* One clinic per week (probably combined with the follow-up ID patient clinic) (6 new, or 15 review or follow-up patients, or in proportion)
- *Patients for review* One clinic per week, possibly combined with new patient clinic
- *Special clinics within the specialty* Usually within the hospital. ID lends itself to the development of specialised services. Diseases such as HIV/AIDS, viral hepatitis, TB and Chronic Fatigue Syndrome can be managed more efficiently along single pathology clinic lines. Academic physicians may wish to develop specialist interest clinics which assist research and improve patient access to new therapies eg new vaccine clinics, HIV research etc)

▪ *General medical clinic*   One combined new and review clinic (6 new patients or 15 review or follow-up patients, or in proportion)

▪ *Telephone consultation*   This can take up to a session per week, as local, regional and national telephone consultations are common.

The general medical clinic commitment would only apply to consultants with a specific commitment to general internal medicine.

Specialised services within the specialty

ID lends itself to such specialised services. Domiciliary antibiotic services are well-developed in some parts of the UK, and some units have highly developed travel clinics, for example. Academic ID and tropical medicine consultants will invariably have such duties, but these should be scaled down in line with the level of their clinical commitment. For the general physician with an ID interest, this will occur only where time, resources, needs and interests permit.

Services outwith the base hospital

▪ *Clinics at other hospitals*   For example, Obstetric units, Hepatology/Gastroenterology units, Genitourinary Medicine units, Respiratory units, paediatric units

▪ *Outreach clinics*   Prisons, homeless shelters, refugee centres, drug dependency

▪ *Domiciliary work*   As required

▪ *Hospice work*   Occasionally, in relation to HIV/AIDS, hepatic cirrhosis, or terminal cancer presenting as part of an ID pathology (eg hepatitis C).

For the general physician with an ID interest or the academic ID physician, this will occur only where time, resources, needs and interests permit.

On-call for specialist advice and emergencies

Specialty-based on-call cover is constant (24 hours per day, seven days per week), with a rota involving all ID consultant staff in the unit. Academic ID consultants will have such on-call duties, and will have to contribute to the out-of-hour on call rota in order to demonstrate continuing ability to function within the specialty of ID. Tropical medicine physicians face similar challenges.

Some geographically adjacent ID Units have cross-cover arrangements between their consultant staff.

2   Work to maintain and improve the quality of care

This work encompasses duties in clinical governance, professional self-regulation, continuing professional development, education and training of others. For many consultants, at various times in their careers, it may include research, serving in management, and providing advice. All require consultant participation. Such work is described fully in Part 1 of Consultant Physicians Working for Patients. Its scope is summarised in the Appendix to Part 2. Management and advisory work are identified specifically in the Appendix.

MEDICAL WORKFORCE REQUIREMENTS OF THE SPECIALTY

CCST-holding consultants

There is approximately one ID consultant (total 60) per 800,000 of the population of England, or one per 610,000 if the 20 tropical medicine specialists are included (although some of these are primarily practising overseas). In Scotland there are 18 ID consultants for a total population of 5 million (1 per 270,000). At least one long-established English medical school has no associated clinical infectious disease specialists although this is shortly to be remedied, and not all of the new medical schools have firm plans to include ID academics. The coverage of different health regions differs widely. International comparisons are difficult, but in Sweden (population 8.9 million) there are about 330 specialists in 30 units (1 per 27,000); in Norway (population 4.5m) there are 74 (1 per 61,000); in the Netherlands (pop 15.8m) there are 52 ID and seven tropical medicine specialists, (ie 1 per 267,000).[17,18] In Australia there is one ID specialist per 174,000 adults.[19] At the other extreme, in the USA (population 256m), 458 consultant level positions in infectious diseases were advertised in 1993 and 340 in 1995.[20] However, the overlap between clinical microbiology and infectious disease is less well defined in North America compared to the UK, where approximately five ID positions are advertised each year.

The true need for ID physicians is difficult to quantify although there is ample evidence that the quality of care that they deliver is better than that delivered by non-specialists.[12,13] By comparison with our Scandinavian and Dutch neighbours and with Australia, a reasonable target in the medium term would be provision of one specialist per 250,000 population, with a further 20–30 in more specialist practice in the academic centres (including tropical medicine), ie 200 specialists in England (pop 50m) on a capitation basis plus 30 extra, or 230 total for England.

This figure equates well with the recent combined Colleges and BMA recommendation that there should be 2–3 infection specialists in each DGH unit serving a population of about 300,000.[15] One of these should be a clinical ID specialist, so for approximately 255 DGH units there is currently the need for 255 specialists in England. A similar recommendation was made in a joint Colleges consultative document over a decade ago[16] and the need is more pressing now than it was then.

▌ *Specialist registrars in training* – to ensure an adequate supply of applicants for consultant posts in ID and Tropical Medicine (including academic Lecturer-specialist registrar posts).

▌ *Staff grade doctors* – to ensure that clinical activity continues at an adequate level of quality (eg involvement in specialist service delivery etc).

▌ *Senior house officers* – to ensure future development of the specialty of ID, and to familiarise doctors intending to work in other areas of medicine with the specialty.

▌ *Junior house officers* – to ensure future development of the specialty of ID, and to familiarise doctors intending to work in other areas of medicine with the specialty.

▌ *Other grades of staff,* such as nurse consultants and nurse practitioners, may influence the exact requirements for medical staffing.

Consultant workforce projections

For the purposes of workforce projections (see Tables 1–6, pp27–32) all ID consultants are presumed to work one WTE, although the majority are academics typically on a maximum 6/11 clinical contract and many of the remainder have time commitments to other specialities especially general internal medicine. Tropical medicine has been included with infectious diseases in the current total of ID specialists in England.

NOTE: *In 1999 there was insufficient information available to allow a more precise estimate of the workforce requirements in this specialty. This recent estimate provides a firmer basis for workforce planning but this too will need to be reviewed in the light of developments in practice and service delivery.*

WORK PROGRAMME FOR A CONSULTANT IN INFECTIOUS DISEASES AND/OR TROPICAL MEDICINE (WITH ADAPTATIONS FOR JOINT WORK WITH GENERAL INTERNAL MEDICINE OR ACADEMIC APPOINTMENTS)

Examples demonstrate three different work patterns, but other permutations are possible. If appropriate allocation of NHDs (as advised by the BMA) were as provided for on-call commitments, the figures below would need substantial downward adjustment.

1 Direct patient care

	Infectious diseases and/or tropical medicine only	Infectious diseases and/or tropical medicine plus GIM	Infectious diseases and/or tropical medicine – academic
Work in the specialty	NHDs	NHDs	NHDs
Inpatient work	3–4	2–3	2
Outpatient clinics	2–3	1–2	1
Specialised investigative and therapeutic procedure clinics	0	0	0
Specialised services	1	0–1	0–1
Work outwith the base hospital	0–1	0–1	0–1
On-call for specialist advice and emergencies	NHDs not allocated	NHDs not allocated	NHDs not allocated
Work in acute medicine			
On-take and mandatory post-take rounds	0	2	0
Outpatient clinics	0	1	0
Work in academic medicine	0	0	5
Total	*6–9*	*5–10*	*8–10*

References

1.   House of Lords Committee. *Resistance to antibiotics and other antimicrobial agents.* London, HMSO Stationery Office 1998.

2.   Standing Medical Advisory Committee of the Department of Health. *The path of least resistance.* Department of Health, 1998.

3.   Nathwani D. A role for an infectious disease physician. *Proc Roy Coll Phys Edin* 1999;**29**:289–292.

4.   McKendrick MW. Clinical infection services – the UK perspective. *Clin Microbiol Infect* 2000;**6**:419–422.

5. Wilkins EG, Hickey MM, Khoo S *et al.* Northwick Park infection consultation service. Part 1. Aims and operation of the service and general distribution of the service between September 1987 and July 1990. *J Infect* 1991;**23**: 47–56.

6. Nathwani D, Davey P, France AJ, *et al.* Impact of an infection consultation service for bacteraemia on clinical management and use of resources. *Q J Med* 1996;**89**:789–797.

7. Fowler VG, Sanders LL, Sexton DJ *et al.* Outcome of *Staphylococcus aureus* bacteremia according to compliance with recommendations of infectious disease specialists. Experience with 244 patients. *Clin Infect Dis* 1998;**27**: 478–486.

8. Byl B, Clevenburgh P, Jacobs F *et al.* Impact of infectious disease specialists and microbiological data on the appropriateness of antimicrobial therapy for bacteremia. *Clin Infect Dis* 1999;**29**:60–66.

9. Cohen J, Roberts C. Joint training programme. *Roy Coll Pathol Bull* 2000;**109**:30–33.

10. Cohen J. Training in infectious diseases – looking to the future. *Clin Microbiol Infect* 2000;**6**:449–452.

11. Beeching NJ, Borysciewicz LK. Training in infectious diseases and tropical medicine in Britain. *Clin Microbiol Infect* 2000;**6**:432–434.

12. Scottish Needs Assessment Programme. *Inpatient resources for communicable diseases in Scotland.* Glasgow: Scottish Forum for Public Health Medicine 1994.

13. Arblaster L. *Continuing to contain the unpredictable: the future for infectious disease expertise.* University of Leeds, Department of Public Health Medicine, 1994.

14. Royal College of Physicians. Consultant physicians working for patients. Part I. A blueprint for effective hospital practice. *J Roy Coll Phys Lond* 1998;**32**(4) Supplement 1:S1–S20.

15. Joint Working Party of BMA, RCP London and RCS England. *Provision of acute general hospital services.* Consultation Document. London: Royal College of Surgeons of England, 1998.

16. Tyrrell DAJ, Banatvala JE, Hurley DR, *et al.* Training in infectious diseases. *J Roy Coll Phys Lond* 1990;**24**: 161–166.

17. McKendrick MW, Beeching NJ. *Survey of European workforce in infection specialities* (in preparation).

18. Bannister B. Infectious diseases: who cares and how much? *J Roy Coll Phys Lond* 1996;**30**:77–79.

19. Dent O. Clinical workforce in internal medicine and paediatrics in Australia 1997. *Fellowship Affairs* (Royal Australasian College of Physicians) Feb 1999;**18**(1):31–46.

20. Preheim LC. Career opportunities for infectious diseases subspecialists. *Clin Infect Dis* 1998;**26**:277–281.

Intensive care medicine

1   The specialty

In June 1999 the Specialist Training Authority granted recognition to the specialty of intensive care medicine (as a dual CCST with anaesthesia, or general internal medicine, or surgery). Such recognition represents accumulation of many years development of the concept of intensive care, which emerged largely as a response to developments in medicine and surgery. Further, in some specialties (particularly neurosciences, cardiac and burns) intensive care units have been developed specifically for patient care within these disciplines. High dependency units have been introduced to provide a step between intensive care and ward care, sometimes in dedicated units and sometimes associated with particular specialties. Overall development has been unplanned and haphazard, and has largely relied upon the interest of local clinicians to develop it. Thus, in March 1999, an expert group was established by the Department of Health to propose a framework for the future organisation and delivery of *adult critical care services*. The group had the remit to produce a national framework for adult critical care services, which is evidence-based (or based upon clear professional consensus) and which sets out operational standards for staffing and transfer levels in intensive care and high dependency units, and makes recommendations for the level, configuration and mix of provision of general adult and neurological adult intensive care and high dependency care services.[1]

The implementation of this report is likely to take in excess of two years and is currently under way. The characteristics of the modernised service will be based upon integration. Thus, a hospital-wide approach to critical care services that extends beyond the physical boundaries of intensive care and high dependency care is envisaged, which will provide support to and interact and communicate with the range of acute services. The service will also be provided in the context of an integrated network involving several trusts working to common standards and protocols, providing a comprehensive range of critical care services. Workforce development is planned (see below) and the service is to be underpinned by good information and a data collection culture promoting an appropriate evidence base.

2   Work of consultants who practise in the specialty

Within a critical care service, it is envisaged that consultant medical staff will have responsibility for directing the overall plan of patient clinical care, direct supervision and teaching of trainee medical staff, internal and organisational (non-clinical) management, and leadership of the service. The breakdown of time spent in each role will be dependent upon the nature of the critical care unit, other consultant and non-consultant medical staffing and upon case-mix, throughput and the range of services provided. The need to oversee or provide informal advice in other acute care areas will also affect the work pattern.

3   Workforce requirements

The medical workforce requirements for critical care are currently unclear. An Audit Commission report[2] noted that less than half the intensive care units in the UK had a consultant presence in the unit on every weekday session. This, and the progressive increase in the size and complexity of intensive care units, will lead to the need for additional manpower. Work is likely to be commissioned to assess the medical workforce needs in the context of the document *Comprehensive critical care*,[1] and not just intensive care medicine.

References

1.   *Comprehensive critical care: a review of adult critical care services.* Department of Health 1999.

2.   *Critical to success. The place of efficient and effective critical care services within the acute hospital.* London: Audit Commission, 1999.

Medical oncology

i   Introduction: a brief description of the specialty

Medical oncologists are physicians who have specialised in the assessment and management of patients with cancer. They are trained to use systemic drugs in the treatment of cancer, and to administer these therapies to patients who either have localised or metastatic malignancy in need of systemic therapy or whose cancer has potentially been cured by surgery but for whom further adjuvant systemic therapy improves their outlook. The role of the medical oncologist is to discuss the treatment options with patients, supervise the therapy and manage any complications of disease and/or treatment that may arise. All such patient management is done in consultation with other clinicians within the context of multidisciplinary meetings and clinical networks.

Some people are confused about the distinction between clinical and medical oncologists. They are the two main medical specialities that actively manage patients with non-haematological malignancy. They often work in partnership, and both give systemic therapy to patients, but only the clinical oncologists administer radiotherapy. However, this simple definition by exclusion hides a number of other differences in work-pattern, approach and focus, which this document clarifies.

ii   Organisation

Primary care

It is very rare for a patient requiring systemic anti-cancer therapy to be managed solely by a general practitioner. While patients receive such treatment they are either exclusively under the care of the hospital or, preferably, in a shared-care protocol. However, close liaison with primary care is important for the pre-emption and management of treatment or disease-related problems. In those patients who are dying from their disease, the general practitioner has an increasingly important role, often in conjunction with palliative care services. Indeed, one of the challenges of the specialty is to keep the primary care services in the loop during the active management phase, so that should it be necessary the transition to a terminal phase of management is easier for both the GP and the patient.

Secondary/tertiary care

As hospital physicians, medical oncologists are based in the secondary and tertiary care system. Most work in large departments, often teaching hospitals. A significant number hold academic posts, but more and more full-time NHS consultants are being appointed. Some are based primarily in DGHs, and others may have a regular clinical commitment to a peripheral hospital. Increasingly medical oncologists are involved in the management of the common solid tumours, supervising and directing systemic therapy in conjunction with clinical oncologists, surgeons and other clinicians in multidisciplinary teams. Some units and clinicians also have tertiary and even quarternary roles, providing specialist advice and patient care for the rarer tumours.

iii   Patterns of referral

Most new patient referrals come from other hospital specialists. For the common solid tumours these are for the most part surgeons, but some patients with lung and gastrointestinal cancers are referred from physicians. Patients may also be jointly managed with a clinical oncologist.

Almost all cases are urgent, and it is rare for there to much of a waiting list for new patients. A small proportion of patients may be referred for a second opinion, or come from fellow oncologists who seek particular expertise.

iv   Ways of working: clinical networks and multidisciplinary clinics

Most medical oncologists work in large departments – cancer centres – and specialise in the management of a few types of cancer. Those based in peripheral units, such as cancer units, may well see and treat patients with a number of different cancers, but may still have one area of particular expertise, according to local circumstances. Academics may either follow a similar site-specialisation pattern, or develop expertise in a treatment area, such as intensive or experimental chemotherapy.

It is essential that patients are managed through managed clinical networks, so that geographical differences in treatment options are avoided. Ideally patients will be discussed in multidisciplinary teams, involving surgeons, physicians, clinical and medical oncologists, palliative care specialists, pathologists, and radiologists.

The role of the medical oncologist is not necessarily to see all patients in need of systemic therapy themselves, but they should be involved in the decisions made about appropriate therapeutic options. In addition, most medical oncologists working in multidisciplinary teams play a pivotal role in determining evidence-based treatment protocols, and define research priorities and strategies for the team. At the wider, hospital or regional level, they are often involved in determining NHS Trust and network cancer drug policy.

v   Quality of service

The standard of care delivered to patients with cancer must be consistently high, in order to give patients the best possible outlook. Clinicians should follow agreed national and local guidelines and protocols for treatment. All such guidelines should be evidence based whenever possible. The actual delivery of chemotherapy must be subject to quality controls by both pharmacists and nurses, with regular audit of practice and patient outcome.

The standards that should be set for all areas of activity are set out below.

Referral

All relevant patients should be referred and seen within a reasonable time
Availability of relevant clinico-pathological information
Review of patients within a multidisciplinary network/clinic

Outpatients
Dedicated outpatient clinic area
    Appropriate support nursing and phlebotomy staff
    Appropriate amount of time for new (40 minutes) and review patients (15 minutes)

continued

Sufficient space for relatives to be present during consultation

Access to urgent lab results and radiography

Pharmacy services for dispensing chemotherapy and support drugs

Appropriate secretarial support (both before and after the clinic)

Day-treatment unit for chemotherapy
Dedicated area

Aseptic pharmacy facilities to prepare cytotoxics

Trained nursing staff to administer chemotherapy according to agreed protocols

Facilities for medical assessment of patients before and during chemotherapy

Inpatient beds
Appropriately nursed and resourced beds for treatment of patients

Inpatient chemotherapy for complex regimens

Treatment of complications of disease and therapy

Single room/isolator unit for profoundly neutropenic patients

Access to physiotherapy, occupational therapy and social workers

Access to radiography and laboratory support for emergencies

24-hour on-call consultant cover

Non-consultant ward-based medical staff for day-to-day patient management

Access to ITU, other medical specialities in emergency

Laboratory and other support
Access to laboratory/ other support for in- and outpatient management

Pathology

Haematology

Clinical chemistry

Microbiology

Blood transfusion

Radiology (including interventional)

Physiotherapy

Dietitians

Research infrastructure
This is desirable, but rarely funded by the NHS, more often coming from soft money or cancer charity grants

Research nurse

Data management

Storage facilities for CRFs

Radiology and laboratory support

Local ethical review process

---

vi   Outline of clinical work

The majority of patients are managed as outpatients, both during and after their chemotherapy. The number of clinics per week will vary from unit to unit, but a full-time NHS consultant can expect to do up to four clinics per week. Multidisciplinary clinics and meetings are the foundation of the referral and management patterns, but most patients are likely to be seen in clinics led by one or two medical oncology consultants. Many centres will have chemotherapy or review clinics, where patients are seen each time they attend for therapy, in order to make a brief assessment and prescribe their chemotherapy. Other units provide nurse-led care, so that patients are only seen either when there are problems, or there is a need to make an overall assessment of toxicity and response to therapy. In addition, consultants are expected to do at least one ward round per week, and take part in the general unit activities of audit, management etc. Currently, with most medical oncologists based in cancer centres, there will be specialist registrar trainees to supervise and train.

Research is the cornerstone of medical oncology, which should be evidence-based as much as possible. Given that current anti-cancer therapies leave plenty of scope for improved efficacy, most medical oncologists, whether employed by the NHS or a university/cancer charity, are expected to actively partake in clinical research. This is one of the differentiating features from clinical oncology, a related specialty in which the pattern of work and patient numbers leave less time for an active clinical research programme. It is anticipated therefore that medical oncologists will partake in multi-centre randomised trials, as well as smaller phase II studies, actively recruiting patients from their practice.

vii Work of other members in the team

Clinical nurse specialist

Many units will have a clinical nurse specialist for some tumour sites. Their role includes:

- Discussion with patients the implications of diagnosis
- Ensuring patients are aware of likely toxicities of therapies
- Point of contact for patients to discuss issues relating to disease and/or therapy
- Providing emotional support to outpatients and relatives
- May also help inform patients about clinical trials.

Chemotherapy nurses

These specially trained nurses should administer all in and outpatient chemotherapy.

Research nurses

They may not be present in all units, and their role to some extent will always overlap with clinical nurse specialists. However, their main roles are:

- Recruitment of patients to clinical trials
  - Assessment of patients' eligibility using predefined criteria
  - Further explanation of the process and toxicities of any therapies
  - Co-ordination of trial-related investigations and clinic visits
  - Regular contact with and assessment of patients in trials
  - Administration of experimental therapies
  - Completion of case report forms (not in all units)
- Informing other clinicians/trainees about available trials
- Preparation of data records for monitoring visits (not all units)
- Maintaining a high standard of trial conduct, data and patient level of information.

Pharmacists

- They should supervise the preparation of all chemotherapy.
- They also give advice on drug interactions, and other aspects of chemotherapy.

Clinical oncologists

▌ They are responsible for advising on and supervising any radiotherapy.

▌ Additionally, they usually also supervise the more routine systemic drug therapies.

▌ They provide expertise on therapeutic decision making in multidisciplinary teams.

viii Conjoined services

Medical oncologists need to have access to the following services to assist in the appropriate diagnosis and treatment of their patients:

▌ Surgical oncology

▌ Clinical oncology

▌ Pharmacy

▌ Pathology

▌ Microbiology

▌ Physiotherapy

▌ Radiology

▌ Dietitians.

ix   Specialised facilities

Physical proximity of inpatient and outpatient treatment areas as well as outpatient clinics is desirable. Adequately staffed and resourced units are needed to ensure appropriate levels of care and treatment delivery. Details of these are to be found in section v above.

x   Contribution to acute medicine

Whilst dual accreditation in medical oncology and general internal medicine is possible, very few current medical oncologists also practise acute general medicine, and very few trainees are currently training in both specialties. Future changes in the manner in which training in general internal medicine is carried out and recognised may make dual accreditation easier, but to date there has not been any significant demand for medical oncologists to be dually accredited. It is conceivable that posts based in a district general hospital might be desirous of a consultant who is dually accredited, but the general view of the specialty is that there is sufficient work and expertise required to justify single specialty training and working. This is not to say that there is no general medicine in medical oncology – this could not be further from the truth. Indeed, the title of the Royal College of Physician's document "The cancer patient's physician" reflects the reality that a medical oncologist is required to provide a significant amount of general medical expertise to his/her patients. What medical oncologists should not expect, unless out of their own choice, is to be on the acute general medical on-call rota!

xi   Academic medical oncologists

Academic medical oncologists will have varying NHS workloads. They will usually hold an honorary senior consultant contract, and make a significant contribution to the work of the NHS department. In many units they may share an area of clinical practice with a full-time NHS clinician to provide continuing care, and may sometimes take on a specialist tertiary referral role in the rarer tumours. They will usually have a lighter service workload in order to give more time for research, whether laboratory or clinical, as well as teaching at both undergraduate and post-graduate level. The academic interests can vary from pure clinical to very largely laboratory-based, but there is an increasing trend for many academics to be involved in translational research, with a foot in both the laboratory and clinic!

xii   Future developments to enhance patient care

The national cancer plan for England and Wales envisages an expansion in the number of NHS medical oncologists, which may also be matched by further growth in Scotland. Medical Oncologists will continue to play an increasing role in the delivery of systemic therapy to patients with the common solid tumours, and partake in multidisciplinary discussions for these tumour sites. The development of telemedicine should permit the extension of these discussions to patients managed in peripheral units, since very few cancer units will have sufficient patient numbers to justify visiting oncologists specialising in all major tumour sites.

WORK OF CONSULTANTS IN MEDICAL ONCOLOGY

1   Direct patient care

A Work in the specialty

The measure of a medical oncologist's workload is the number of new patient referrals seen per year. The ideal is 200 per year. This number takes account of the fact that a consultant is not expected to be present 52 weeks a year, but 42 weeks to allow for continuing professional development and holiday. The number of new patients is relatively low because of the prolonged work associated with each individual patient receiving chemotherapy for cancer. Academic medical oncologists have a pro-rata reduction in recognition of their protected time for research and higher teaching commitment, and about 150 new patients per year is more appropriate for them. However, due in large part to the low number of specialist oncologists in much of the UK, the workload of the majority of medical oncologists exceeds these figures.

Inpatient work

In common with clinical oncology, as well as many other medical specialities, the majority of patients are managed and treated as outpatients, with most admissions being for the treatment of complications of either disease or therapy. There are still some chemotherapy regimens that are required to be given as an inpatient, such as some of those including cisplatin or ifosphamide.

Ward rounds with junior staff and ward-based nurses:

- May include other health care workers
    - fellow oncologist
    - microbiologist
    - specialist nurse
    - palliative care team member
- Management of patients with chemotherapy toxicities (e.g. neutropenic sepsis)
- Management of patients with intensive inpatient regimens
- Management of patients with severe disease complications
    - Pleural effusions
    - Hypercalcaemia
    - Severe pain, nausea etc.
- Teaching and training are important components of ward rounds

Referral work of inpatients under other specialties

Outpatient work

The exact organisation of the different classes of patients will vary between one unit and another, and any member of the multidisciplinary team may also undertake the follow-up of potentially cured patients. Some clinics are done with, or in parallel with, other oncologists or members of the multidisciplinary teams.

New patients are usually seen in multidisciplinary and/or specialised oncology clinics:

▯ Usually referred from a surgeon, hospital physician or fellow oncologist

▯ Case may have been previously discussed at pathology or multidisciplinary meeting

▯ 40 minutes per new patient

▯ Some new patients seen first by juniors with subsequent discussion for training.

Review patients:

▯ Second visit to confirm treatment plans and/or get consent for such therapy

▯ Review visit for assessment of treatment response

▯ Follow-up visit for patient off active therapy

▯ Follow-up visit for patient who has been potentially cured
　　surveillance for complications of therapy
　　surveillance for evidence of relapse.

Chemotherapy clinic patients (when not reviewed by day ward nurse-led service):

▯ Patient seen at each chemotherapy dose (usually 3 or 4 weekly)

▯ Checking of full blood count and relevant biochemistry tests

▯ Completion of prescription for chemotherapy

All clinics will require support clerical and nursing staff. The presence of a phlebotomist and site-related clinical nurse specialist are highly desirable.

Services outwith the base hospital

The need to provide these will depend on the local arrangements between cancer centres and units. In many places, medical oncologists are expected to do at least one peripheral clinic, and may well also be required to review inpatients and provide cover for day-case chemotherapy. It would be exceptional for a consultant to have admitting rights with concomitant inpatient responsibility at a peripheral hospital if it is only visited once or twice a week. Therefore arrangements must be in place to provide back-up cover and protocols for the urgent treatment of patients admitted to a peripheral unit. One of the commonest models is that an identified clinician, sometimes a haematologist, takes responsibility for complications arising from the administration of chemotherapy.

On-call work

It is usual for the medical oncologists to partake in a rota to provide 24-hour emergency cover for their own patients. In some centres, especially when there are very few medical oncologists, the rota is shared with the clinical oncologists, but in this case additional cover must be provided for any urgent radiotherapy, since medical oncologists are not expected to be able to prescribe radiotherapy.

The level of work expected during on-call will vary, depending on volume of routine work and the junior staff working. In some units oncology patients are managed by general medical SHOs, whose knowledge of oncology will be such that the consultant may need to get involved in many emergency admissions. More commonly there will be Specialist Registrars training in Medical Oncology, so that the level of consultant work on-call is much less, being confined to perhaps a ward round at the weekend and telephone advice for the difficult cases.

B Acute medicine

Medical oncologists are rarely directly involved in the delivery of care in general internal medicine (but see above).

C Academic medicine

Medical oncologists with academic contracts should not expect to devote more than 6 sessions to NHS service work if their academic work is to flourish. Ideally clinical and academic activities should be complementary.

2 Work to maintain and improve the quality of care

This work encompasses duties in clinical governance, professional self-regulation, continuing professional development, education and training of others. For many consultants, at various times in their careers, it may include research, serving in management, and providing advice. All require consultant participation. Such work is described fully in Part 1 of this document. Its scope is summarised in the Appendix to Part 2. Management and advisory work are identified specifically in the Appendix.

WORKFORCE REQUIREMENTS FOR MEDICAL ONCOLOGY

In November 2000 there were 138 medical oncologists in the UK, and the figure had been rising by about 12% per year over the previous few years. Allowing for university appointments, this equates to 110 whole time equivalent (WTE) posts. Many radiotherapy centres still have no medical oncologists, although plans are underway to fund and advertise posts in some of these centres. Based on current workloads, the ideal number of new patients per consultant, and the best practice of multidisciplinary working, it is recommended that there should be 1.25 WTE medical oncologist per 200,000–250,000 population.[1] It is envisaged that it may take until 2006 to achieve this, since it requires a total of around 300 medical oncologists across the UK, a considerable expansion from the position at the start of the third millennium. In terms of the balance of clinical and medical oncologists, the recent accepted recommendation of the Joint Collegiate Council for Oncology is a ratio of 2:1,[2] and to achieve this figure there would also need to be a significant expansion from the current position.

NOTE: *In 1999 there was insufficient information available to allow a more precise estimate of the workforce requirements in this specialty. This recent estimate provides a firmer basis for workforce planning but this too will need to be reviewed in the light of developments in practice and service delivery.*

References

1. *The cancer patient's physician. Recommendations for the development of medical oncology in England and Wales.* Royal College of Physicians, 2000.

2. *Recommendations for the deployment of clinical and medical oncologists within cancer networks.* Joint Collegiate Council for Oncology (JCCO), 2001.

Neurology

i   Introduction

Clinical neurology is the medical speciality that is concerned with the diagnosis, treatment and – in some instances – continuing assessment and care of patients with diseases of the central nervous system, peripheral nervous system and muscles. For some patients the neurologist is the principal provider of specialist care, but for a much larger number care is provided in collaboration with other physicians and surgeons. Neurologists also play a part in undergraduate and postgraduate education, research and audit, and in service planning.

In addition to patient care and teaching, academic neurologists are required to promote research. This often involves co-operation with other researchers, at national and international levels, with the consequence that they are not always available to perform routine clinical duties. Academic neurologists have a responsibility to teach neurology to undergraduates and postgraduates. Although it is necessary for academic neurologists to have clinical responsibilities, these have to be less than is usual for other neurologists.

Patients referred to neurologists may have straightforward disorders or they may have complex conditions. Overall, 16 common disorders account for 75% of all new patients. The remaining 25% have more unusual disorders, which may require expert assessment, sophisticated investigations and elaborate treatment.

ii   Organisation of clinical services

Within the UK, specialist neurological care is given by consultant neurologists, who are based either at regional or other neurological centres or at district general hospitals (DGHs). Those based at a neuroscience centre provide a local service from the centre and at neighbouring DGHs. Those who are based at a DGH, see patients at a DGH and they may provide a service to other DGHs in the area. All neurologists should be attached to a neuroscience centre because the quality of patient care depends upon this attachment.

Regional and other neuroscience centres

Neuroscience centres are crucial to the provision of high quality care. They should be staffed by neurologists, neurosurgeons, clinical neurophysiologists, neuroradiologists, neuropathologists and other specialist staff and should be provided with all the relevant modern investigative equipment. The centres act as a venue for the integration of specialists with the neurosciences. The availability of all the neuroscience specialties at centres creates the environment essential for the management of the more common disorders and of the less common and more complex conditions that often require a multidisciplinary input.

Much of the continuing medical education of neurologists, and of clinicians in related disciplines takes place at the centres. They also constitute the main focus for undergraduate teaching of neurology, postgraduate education of trainee neurologists and clinical neurological research.

District General Hospitals

Provision for the care of inpatients at the DGH is desirable, but not obligatory. Local circumstances determine the best site for neurology beds. If local support services are adequate, then DGH neurology beds are provided. Where beds are available and the facilities and staffing are adequate, an on-call service for the admission of neurological emergencies can be introduced.

iii   General considerations/workforce requirements/acute neurology

The general characteristics of all consultant neurologist posts should conform to the following:

A   It is the policy of the Association of British Neurologists (ABN) that there should be at least one whole-time equivalent consultant neurologist for every 100,000 population.[1,2] The ABN has recently produced a document aimed at improving the care of patients with acute neurological illness.[3] This states that ward referrals should be seen within twenty-four hours if necessary. Six to seven hundred consultant neurologists are required to begin to provide this more comprehensive service. A consultant expansion of 7% pa would be required to achieve this by 2011 and would represent one neurologist per 85-100,000 population. At present there is a shortage of SpRs applying for consultant posts. Thirty to forty SpRs will receive CSST certificates annually for the next three years. It is highly likely that there needs to be a small increase in the number of neurological SpRs if the current expansion in neurological consultants is to be met, and an improved service offered to both inpatients and outpatients.

B   Consultant neurologists should not be isolated. Wherever possible within a particular geographical area, each neurologist should have at least one colleague, and should also be attached to a specified neuroscience centre.

C   Every neurologist should have a base hospital, where most clinical and other duties are done. The base hospital may be a DGH or a neuroscience centre. In addition, to working at the base hospital, many neurologists will be expected to work at one or at most, two other hospitals. The number of additional hospitals at which a neurologist can be expected to work is determined according to the following principles:

-    Each DGH should be able to identify its own neurologists, who may be based at that DGH, at a neighbouring DGH or at the neuroscience centre. The commitment at a particular DGH should allow urgent referrals to be seen within 24 hours.

-    If a DGH is served by a single neurologist, then that neurologist should have regular clinical commitments at no more than two hospitals, one of which is the base hospital.

-    Some DGHs may be served by two or more neurologists who share the workload, thereby ensuring continuity of cover during absence.

iv   Facilities and services

All consultant neurologists should have ready access for all of the facilities and services listed below. Furthermore, access to such areas should be equal for all neurologists in a given area. Contracts should be prepared to ensure that DGH-based neurologists have just as ready access to these services as centre-based neurologists, although it may not be possible for DGH-based neurologists to safely manage inpatients in the neuroscience centre without a system of shared care. Existing posts where such access is limited should be modified accordingly, and new posts must have such access built into the job description. There should be no exceptions.

▌ *Beds:* An adequate number of beds at the neuroscience centre and at the DGH should be allocated, and protected from use by any other disciplines. Local needs will determine whether they are sited at the neuroscience centre, the DGH or both.

▌ *Junior medical staff:* The minimum requirements are described later in this document, when job plans are given for each type of neurologist. It is imperative that dedicated time from junior staff is allocated to neurology and is not eroded by pressures from other clinical services.

▌ *Secretarial support:* Each consultant neurologist should have a full-time secretary at the base hospital with access to part-time secretarial help at any other hospitals at which clinical duties are performed.

▌ *Specialist nurses:* Specialist nurses, especially those with interests in epilepsy, Parkinson's disease and multiple sclerosis, are important to complement the services provided by medical staff.

▌ *Neurosurgery:* There should be easy access to neurosurgical services, although these do not necessarily have to be in the hospital where the consultant neurologist is based.

▌ *Neurophysiology:* A full consultant-led neurophysiology service should be available to each neurologist. It should not be assumed that the consultant neurologist will do all the neurophysiology.

▌ *Neuroradiology:* There should be ready access to consultant-led neuroradiology services, which should include CT and MRI scanning, angiography and myelography.

▌ *Neuropathology:* There should be ready access to consultant-led neuropathological services, both for muscle and nerve biopsy studies and for post-mortem studies.

▌ *Neuropsychology:* There should be ready access by all neurologists to a neuropsychology service.

▌ *Rehabilitation services:*

　– There should be ready access to rehabilitation facilities and services. These should include physiotherapy, occupational therapy, speech therapy, appliance fitting, clinical psychology, medical social worker and dietician.

　– If the consultant neurologist has expertise and an interest in neurological rehabilitation, he may play a part in providing rehabilitation services provided that specific clinical sessions and resources are allocated for this purpose. It should not be assumed that the consultant neurologist will provide a general rehabilitation service for patients who do not have a neurological disorder.

　– There should be ready access to a Young Disabled Unit which may provide rehabilitation and continuing care. It should not be assumed that the consultant neurologist will supervise such a service without appropriate time being set aside in the timetable and without appropriate resources being provided.

Other facilities

There should also be ready access to neuropsychiatric, pain relief and clinical genetics services. There should also be available specific treatment modalities such as plasma exchange, epilepsy surgery and botulinum toxin treatment.

Future developments

It is appreciated that full implementation of these recommendations will require increased numbers of neurological consultant staff, especially if neurologists are going to play a more important role in the care of common neurological emergencies in future. To illustrate this, the provision of an emergency admitting service for patients with acute neurological disorders requires at least three consultant neurologists and adequate junior staff cover.

WORK OF CONSULTANT NEUROLOGISTS[4]

In the paragraphs that follow, a session is defined as a period of $3\frac{1}{2}$ hours (or one NHD), during which all the activities connected with that session should be completed. These activities include all clinical work, correspondence, travelling and other relevant duties. Fixed commitments are regular scheduled NHS activities that substantially affect the use of NHS resources, such as other staff or facilities. Fixed commitments are those which consultants are required to fulfil, except in emergency or with local management's agreement.

1   Patient care

A Work in the specialty

Inpatient service

Specific NHDs should be allocated for seeing ward referrals; 1–2 such NHDs should be in the job description.

Outpatient service

The timetable should not contain more than three fixed outpatient NHDs in a week. One of these may be a special interest clinic. Other outpatient NHDs may be performed if that is the wish of the neurologist, but these must not be regarded as fixed.

A *new patient* is regarded as a patient not seen before; or a patient who was discharged from the outpatient clinic or ward one year or more prior to the date of the clinic: or an old patient with a new complaint. An *old patient* is a person who is a regular attender as a *follow-up patient* or one who was discharged from the clinic or ward less than a year prior to the date of the clinic session.

A reasonable outpatient workload depends on the case mix and the number, seniority and experience of doctors in attendance. The time allocated to new and old patients should be calculated by the consultant, and the number of patients should be adhered to by clinic staff. The quality of care in the outpatient clinic much depends upon the time available for each patient and should not be compromised. Supervision of junior staff and teaching undergraduates takes time. The following is a guide to the ideal time expenditure for each neurological outpatient.

- New patient: 30 min for a consultant
                                40 min for registrar
- Follow-up patient: 15 min for a consultant
                                20 min for a registrar
- An extra 25% of these times should be allowed for the teaching of medical students, or when inexperienced junior staff require close supervision.

Subspecialty services

Many consultant neurologists perform subspeciality clinics. These include services for epilepsy, multiple sclerosis, Parkinson's disease and the movement disorders (including botulinum toxin clinics), vascular disease, dementia, headache, neurogenetics, neuromuscular disorders and motor neurone disease. Such subspecialisation is to be encouraged. It also has the full support of the patient charities.

On-call for neurological emergencies

On-call duties should not exceed one in three.

2 Work to maintain and improve the quality of care

This work encompasses duties in clinical governance, professional self-regulation, continuing professional development, education and training of others. For many consultants, at various times in their careers, it may include research, serving in management, and providing advice. All require consultant participation. Such work is described fully in Part 1 of this document. Its scope is summarised in the Appendix to Part 2. Management and advisory work are identified specifically in the Appendix.

ACADEMIC NEUROLOGISTS

Nature of the appointment

An academic post may be funded by a university, the Medical Research Council (MRC), the NHS, a charity or by a combination of these resources. The appointment should be within a university department of clinical neuroscience and based at a regional centre.

Types of contract

Irrespective of the sources of funding, an academic appointee will hold a paid contract with a university or the MRC. It is usually a condition of clinical academic contracts that the consultant also holds a contract with the NHS to allow access to patients for teaching and research.

The majority of academic consultants in neurology in the UK hold a full-time university or MRC contract (ie the full-time salary is paid by the university or MRC), and an Honorary (unpaid) contract with the NHS. The honorary NHS contract should usually cover six NHDs. The holding of a concurrent full-time university contract accepts that activities carried out during NHS duties are irrelevant to the performance of teaching and research.

An alternative type of contract, known as an A+B contract, is one in which the consultant is employed part-time by the university or MRC for a specified number of NHDs paid by the university or MRC and part-time on an NHS contract for the remainder of the NHDs paid by the NHS. On appointment at Senior Lecturer level, A+B contracts should usually specify five university NHDs and six NHS NHDs, but the balance may need to be altered to allow for academic promotion. A+B contracts can also employ the academic consultant jointly on a whole-time basis with both the university or MRC and the NHS.

National Health Service – clinical duties

The job plan for an academic neurologist should have no more than three fixed NHDs (50% of the NHS workload) as a part of the National Health Service contract. Because the duties of an academic neurologist are different from those of other types of neurologist, the rules on fixed clinical NHDs should be interpreted with much greater flexibility.

The number of fixed commitments should be agreed by the consultant and the management in consultation with the Dean and/or Head of Department. To allow flexibility, it may be practical in some institutions for the contract to state the number of fixed NHDs to be covered by the academic unit as a whole, rather than by specified individuals.

The clinical duties should be at a single neuroscience centre, with any additional duties at no more than one district general hospital. The sessions of clinical duties should not exceed:

Outpatient clinics – 2 NHDs
Ward rounds – 2 NHDs
Attendance at postgraduate meetings – 1 NHD
Administration, travelling, on-call – 1 NHD
(See Table (i))

If the academic neurologist is attached to a DGH, then NHDs for outpatients and ward opinions should be undertaken from those defined above. The Health Authority or Trust that administers the DGH should pay for the relevant NHDs at the DGH and associated travelling expenses.

University – academic duties

The academic contracts should include responsibilities for research, administration and undergraduate teaching of neurology. Postgraduate teaching of neurology should be seen as part of the NHS contract.

Junior staff

Within a university department at a regional neuroscience centre, there should be trainees in neurology at specialist registrar level, and there should be an adequate number of senior house officers.

NEUROSCIENCE-BASED NEUROLOGISTS

Centre-based neurologists spend the majority of their time at neuroscience centres. Attachments to DGHs should conform to the principles outlined earlier. At least 2 NHDs should be spent at the DGH, one of which should be a fixed NHD. The remaining NHDs should be at the centre.

The contract for a centre-based neurologist should contain no more than 6 fixed NHDs per week, of which not more than 3 should be at outpatients.

Special interest or research outpatient clinics may be included in the 3 fixed outpatient NHDs or as an extra, according to the wishes of the consultant.

The remaining duties should be regarded by employing authorities as non-fixed NHDs. The Health Authority or Trust that administers the DGH should pay for the relevant NHDs and associated travelling expenses. Employing authorities must not regard such NHDs at DGHs as commitments that can be dispensed with.

Junior staff

With a neuroscience centre there should be trainees in neurology at specialist registrar level and there should be adequate number of senior house officers.

DGH-BASED NEUROLOGISTS

DGH-based neurologists spend most of their time at the DGH. They should visit their neuroscience centre for an absolute minimum of 2 NHDs per week with proper consideration of travelling time. Their contract should contain no more than 6 *fixed NHDs* of which not more than 3 should be at outpatients.

The health authority or trust that administers the DGH where the neurologist is based should pay for the relevant NHDs and associated travelling expenses. Employing authorities must not regard visits to the Centre as commitments that can be dispensed with.

Junior staff

Within a department of neurology at a DGH, it is reasonable for there to be trainees in neurology at specialist registrar level.

WORKFORCE REQUIREMENTS FOR NEUROLOGY

(See also iii above.) In 2000, there were 350 consultants in this specialty in the UK, or 1 per 155,000 of the population. The number of consultants needed to provide a high quality service in neurology nationally has been estimated as 1 per 100,000 of the population; this equates to 500–600 consultant neurologists. The number of neurologists will almost certainly need to increase further if a more active part is taken in caring for acute neurological illness; the required minimum would then be 700 consultants.

NOTE: *In 1999 there was insufficient information available to allow a more precise estimate of the workforce requirements in this specialty. This recent estimate provides a firmer basis for workforce planning but this too will need to be reviewed in the light of developments in practice and service delivery.*

WORK PROGRAMME

The following examples of work programmes summarise the work of consultant neurologists in a number of settings, giving the recommended workload, and allocation of notional half days (NHDs).

(i) Example of the work programme of consultant physicians in neurology, based in an academic centre, as notional half days (NHDs) per week.

Activity	Workload	NHDs
Patient care		
Ward rounds[1]		2
Outpatient clinics[1]		2
New patients	6 patients per session or	
Follow-up patients	15 patients per session	
Work to maintain and improve the quality of care		2–6

Total: The number of NHDs worked by a consultant can be very variable. Most work programmes indicate an excess of 10 units worked. Obviously, there will be times in the career of a consultant when management and national duties will be carried out to increase the number of NHDs.

[1] Normally some are fixed each week.
Formal teaching is normally at fixed times.

(ii) Example of the work programme of consultant physicians in neurology, based in a district general hospital, as notional half days (NHDs) per week.

Activity	Workload	NHDs
At the DGH		
Patient care		
Ward rounds[1]		2
Ward referrals		2
Outpatient clinics[1]		2
New patients	6 patients per session or	
Follow-up patients	15 patients per session	
Work to maintain and improve the quality of care		2
At the centre		
Outpatient clinics		Minimum of 2
Attendance at postgraduate meetings		
Audit		
Specialist services		
Discussion on patients/investigations		

Total: The number of NHDs worked by a consultant can be very variable. Most work programmes indicate an excess of 10 units worked. Obviously, there will be times in the career of a consultant when management and national duties will be carried out to increase the number of NHDs.

[1] Normally some are fixed each week
Formal teaching is normally at fixed times

(iii) Example of the work programme of consultant physicians in neurology, based in a neurosciences centre, as notional half days (NHDs) per week.

Activity	Workload	NHDs
At the centre		
Patient care		
Ward rounds and inpatient work[1]		
Ward referrals		2
Outpatient clinics[1]		1–2
New patients	6 patients per session or	
Follow-up patients	15 patients per session	
Specialist services		variable
On-call duties		variable
Work to maintain and improve the quality of care		2–4
At the DGH		
Patient care		
Ward rounds and inpatient work[1]		0.5
Ward referrals		
Advice on emergencies		variable
Outpatient clinics[1]		1–2
New patients	6 patients per session or	
Follow-up patients	15 patients per session	
Work to maintain and improve the quality of care		0.5

Total: The number of NHDs worked by a consultant can be very variable. Most work programmes indicate an excess of 10 units worked. Obviously, there will be times in the career of a consultant when management and national duties will be carried out to increase the number of NHDs.

Note: See paper for fuller guidance.
[1] Normally some are fixed each week
Formal teaching is normally at fixed times.

References

1. *Neurology in the United Kingdom: Compiled by numbers of clinical neurologists and trainees.* Compiled on behalf of the Association of British Neurologists by David L Stevens, 1996.

2. *Neurology in the United Kingdom: Towards 2000 and beyond.* Association of British Neurologists. 1997.

3. *Neurology in the United Kingdom: Good neurological practice with particular reference to job plans for consultant neurologists.* Association of British Neurologists. 1993; revised 1998.

4. *Care of acute neurological emergencies.* Association of British Neurologists. 2001 (in preparation).

Nuclear medicine

i   Introduction

Nuclear medicine comprises all applications of radioactive materials in diagnosis, therapy and research, with the exception of the use of sealed radiation sources in radiotherapy.[1] The range and complexity of diagnostic investigations has increased considerably in recent years, reflecting both continuing radiopharmaceutical development and the wider availability of tomographic cameras. Advances in drug radiolabelling and delivery systems have led to a parallel expansion in unsealed source therapy, extending the range of conditions that can be treated by this approach. The rising importance of positron emission tomography using dedicated scanners or by adaptation of gamma cameras will have a major impact upon future workload patterns.

ii   Organisation

Nuclear medicine services are hospital based. Provision varies according to the size and case mix of the population served and reflects the degree of centralisation of nuclear medicine services within individual hospitals. In some centres, nuclear medicine is directed from one specialist department, while in others, the service is delivered by individual practitioners responsible for a specific clinical area.

Service delivery varies between hospitals of different types.[2] Small departments undertaking a limited range of diagnostic investigations follow an outpatient clinic model and are often organised within departments of radiology. Larger centres offering a comprehensive range of imaging, non-imaging diagnostic procedures and unsealed source therapy require day care and dedicated inpatient facilities.

Some areas have developed a hub and spoke model of provision comprising a large department, often within a teaching hospital, linked to a number of local district general hospitals. Specialist services and inpatient facilities are provided in the central unit and consultants undertake sessions in central and outreach hospitals.

Consultants with particular expertise may receive tertiary referrals from other centres for specific procedures such as positron emission tomography, specialist tumour imaging or therapeutic procedures.

iii   Ways of working, clinical networks

Nuclear medicine is a multidisciplinary specialty comprising physicians, radiologists, nurses, physicists, radiographers, pharmacists, clinical scientists and medical laboratory technicians. Local circumstances, particularly the level of overall clinical support within departments dictate regular clinical commitments to sub-specialist areas such as nuclear cardiology, endocrinology and paediatrics. Most nuclear medicine specialists undertake radionuclide therapy and may be the lead clinicians in joint clinics for the management of benign and malignant disease.

Nuclear medicine specialists liaise with a range of other specialties, particularly radiology, oncology, cardiology, neurology, nephrology, paediatrics, orthopaedics and endocrinology. Participation in cross specialty meetings is valuable for cost effective service provision.

iv   Quality

The definition of explicit service standards provides a framework for improving patient care. Generic quality guidelines for the provision of radionuclide imaging services have been developed in the UK by the British Nuclear Medicine Society.[3] These cover aspects of clinical effectiveness, safety and timeliness and include explicit recommendations on appropriate facilities, equipment, staffing, administration, referral prioritisation, performance and reporting of investigations. The guidelines offer a structure for the contracting process and for peer review organisational audit.

v   Clinical governance

The delivery of nuclear medicine services in departments where there is no sessional commitment to nuclear medicine or where departments undertake very few studies has implications for service quality and clinical governance. The situation is compounded in some centres by dividing a limited nuclear medicine caseload between a large number of consultants, diluting individual experience.[4]

Single-handed specialists working independently cannot easily fulfil the requirements of clinical governance. A minimum 0.4 WTE consultant overlap with single-handed practices is encouraged to avoid clinical isolation. In some cases this may be achieved by ensuring the single-handed practitioner rotates to another unit as part of their weekly commitment. The potential role of telemedicine links with larger centres should be explored.

vi   Outline of clinical work in the specialty

Nuclear medicine specialists are responsible for the selection, supervision and reporting of diagnostic investigations, administration of unsealed source therapy and provision of appropriate follow-up. Subspecialist areas include nuclear cardiology, oncology, metabolic bone disease and paediatrics.

Clinicians with a significant radionuclide therapy workload will have fixed sessions for outpatient clinics and inpatient ward rounds and treatment administration. Cross-specialty liaison within the framework of joint clinics for the management of complex malignancy requires further development.

vii   Multidisciplinary teamwork

Non-medical personnel are essential to routine nuclear medicine service provision. Staffing arrangements vary between departments, but may include:

- Nuclear medicine nurses, including nurse practitioners
- Radiographers
- Medical technical officers

▌ Physicists

▌ Clinical scientists

▌ Medical laboratory scientific officers, and

▌ Pharmacists.

Play specialists and cardiac technicians may contribute to specialist services in centres with a high paediatric or cardiac case mix.

viii Specialist facilities

Outpatient investigations

▌ Dedicated patient waiting area

▌ Separate radiopharmaceutical administration area

▌ Examination room

▌ Radiopharmaceutical storage area

▌ Image analysis area

▌ Data reporting room

▌ Educational and library area

▌ Separate paediatric waiting/play area, where appropriate

▌ Access to cardiac stress testing, where appropriate.

Inpatient unit

Inpatient unsealed source therapy must take place in a dedicated facility complying with all statutory requirements for radiation protection, staffed by appropriately trained nurses and physics personnel. Therapy rooms should have individual shower and toilet facilities.

There is a current shortfall in provision of inpatient unsealed source therapy beds in the UK. Published survey data of 20 European countries highlight wide variations in access to isolation facilities.[5] In 1999, 1520 isolation beds were available for a population of 478 million, giving a mean provision of one bed per 286,000 population. At present, the UK provides one bed per 667,000, which is inadequate to meet existing workload pressures within acceptable waiting times. A substantial increase in bed provision is required urgently to match predicted demand for new unsealed source treatments. The proposed expansion of nuclear medicine services within cancer centres will provide opportunities for closer cross specialty liaison and the shared use of purpose built, shielded facilities should be encouraged to ensure cost effective room occupancy.

THE WORK OF CONSULTANTS IN NUCLEAR MEDICINE

The workload of nuclear medicine specialists covers a broad spectrum ranging from reporting routine *in vitro* studies to complex tomographic imaging and radionuclide therapy. Workload estimates must balance the time element required for procedures grouped by type and allow for variations between consultants. The latter reflects the provision for delegation and overall support within, for example, nursing, physics and technical staff.

1 Direct patient care

Workload

The workload figures proposed are based upon the time taken to undertake completed procedures, including:

i   clinical vetting and discussion of referrals

ii reviewing patient data to confirm that procedures are of a satisfactory technical standard.

> This may involve discussion with other professional staff or with individual patients, reporting clinical data and reviewing clinical notes or other imaging

iii checking the written report.

No account has been taken of interruptions that might reduce efficiency. Further adjustments may be required where individual consultants are responsible for administering radio-pharmaceuticals and monitor or oversee work delegated to others. The additional time commitment to sub-specialist areas such as cardiac stress testing or paediatric imaging should be considered separately.

Basis for estimating the time required to complete individual procedures

Procedures have been considered in categories according to complexity. The times listed below are approximations reached by consensus between consultants working in departments of different types. It is assumed that figures will allow a balance to be achieved between straightforward reports and those requiring more detailed assessment. Further details of the analysis are listed separately in the Appendix (p203).

	Time (min)
Routine *in vitro* studies, planar imaging and bone densitometry	10
Complex tomographic imaging	15
Image co-registration studies	30
Positron emission tomography	45
Therapy	
Outpatient therapy: New patient	45
Follow-up	20
Inpatient therapy:	Variable according to length of patient stay

2 Work to maintain and improve the quality of care

Teaching and training

Nuclear medicine is a multidisciplinary specialty. In addition to undergraduate and postgraduate teaching, nuclear medicine consultants will have substantial training commitments to non-medical staff including physicists, radiographers, technicians and specialist nurses. The time commitment to structured Specialist Registrar training, including documentation and performance appraisal should be considered separately.

Continuing medical education, clinical audit and clinical governance

Consultants are expected to spend at least 50 hours per annum on continuing medical education. Formal participation in interdisciplinary meetings is a requirement for good clinical practice and additional time should be allowed for informal clinical consultation. The work plan should include protected time for clinical audit, which will often be undertaken at regional or national level. Provision may be required for some consultants to undertake a lead role in clinical governance.

Research

Nuclear medicine techniques are used extensively in medical research. All consultants are expected to take an active interest in research although the time commitment to this activity will vary according to individual interest and hospital type.

Administration

This includes correspondence, waiting list management, record keeping and tasks undertaken with the support of secretarial staff. Work related to complaints and litigation procedures might be included.

Management

Many nuclear medicine consultants have managerial duties as heads of department and budget holders and undertake appraisal of medical staff. Protected time is necessary for departmental and directorate meetings. Clinical service directors may have responsibility for service planning, requiring additional time allocation. Nuclear medicine consultants have unique legal responsibilities with respect to Administration of Radioactive Substances Advisory Committee (ARSAC) certification for all diagnostic, therapy and research procedures.

Off-site duties and committee work

The small number of nuclear medicine consultants nationally results in an unusually strong commitment to external duties relating to educational and professional issues. Adequate provision for local and off-site managerial duties and committee work should be included in the job plan.

The time commitment to supporting activities has been extrapolated from a published model.[2] As this aspect of workload varies according to local circumstances and hospital type, considerable variation between individual consultants is expected. The following data are for general guidance only and can be applied flexibly to meet local requirements:

	NHDs per week
Small DGH	1
Medium DGH	4
Large DGH	4
Small TH	5
Large TH	5

Definitions[2]

Small DGH	1 camera; 1,500 investigations p.a.
Medium DGH	2 cameras; 2,400 investigations + *in vitro* + therapy
Large DGH	2+ cameras; 5,000 investigations + *in vitro* + therapy
Small TH	2+ cameras; 5,000 investigations + *in vitro* + therapy
Large TH	3+ cameras; 7–10,000 investigations + *in vitro* + therapy

WORKFORCE REQUIREMENTS FOR CONSULTANTS IN NUCLEAR MEDICINE

The above figures can be applied to identify the total annual workload of individual consultants. In practice, this will vary according to the number of contracted NHDs, hospital type and degree of sub-specialisation.

Review of consultant job plans for an individual department will give a realistic indication of the workload that the consultant group should be undertaking within their contracted NHDs. Correlation with annual patient attendance data will also identify the increase in consultant establishment required to manage the caseload.

National nuclear medicine consultant staffing

The 1996/97 South Thames Nuclear Medicine Survey indicated 1.3 whole time equivalent nuclear medicine consultants per one million population.[6] Extrapolation to the total UK population of 58 million would give 76 fulltime nuclear medicine consultants. The Survey data did not allow an assessment of the provision of medical sessions free from other commitments. Taken with a significant increase in procedure complexity over the past five years, this figure underestimates reasonable staffing levels. The European average value is 3.6 consultants per 1m population.[7] Translated to the UK population, this would require 232 consultants.

A realistic figure of 200 nuclear medicine consultants in the UK is proposed, each consultant serving a population of around 300,000.

Retirement planning

Two recent surveys of manpower and related training issues[4,8] predict between 100 and 120 retirements within 10 years. Approximately 50% of replacements will need to be fully trained in all aspects of nuclear medicine (ie imaging, non-imaging and therapy procedures). This level of replacement is unsustainable within existing training numbers.

Over 200 individuals are listed on the nuclear medicine specialist register, of whom only a minority hold a CCST in nuclear medicine. The majority of those registered do not work exclusively in nuclear medicine and it is difficult to estimate the number of new posts that will eventually be necessary to meet proposed standards. It is likely that some retiring staff currently have no identified sessions to perform nuclear medicine but will need to be replaced by fully trained clinicians. This will lead to an expansion of absolute consultant numbers, which will need to be justified to trusts. All trusts will need to identify specific sessional allocation to their existing nuclear medicine services and should be alerted to potential anomalies in current service provision.

NOTE: *In 1999 there was insufficient information available to allow a more precise estimate of the workforce requirements in this specialty. This recent estimate provides a firmer basis for workforce planning but this too will need to be reviewed in the light of developments in practice and service delivery.*

Service delivery

Survey data indicate that some Trusts are only performing a small number of non-imaging nuclear medicine procedures annually, raising questions of service quality. Taken with predicted manpower shortages outlined above, an urgent review of nuclear medicine service delivery in the UK is under consideration.

A hub and spoke model is proposed, based upon the existing cancer centre framework.[9] It is recommended that priority be given to ensuring nuclear medicine specialist support for all UK cancer centres. Central (hub) functions would include imaging, non-imaging tests and unsealed source therapy for benign and malignant disease. Smaller departments (spoke) will undertake radionuclide imaging and therapy for benign disease, where appropriate.

It is likely that PET facilities will be organised within the cancer centre framework and that further consultant expansion will be required to meet this development.

WORK PROGRAMME

In clinical practice it is usual to schedule procedures by type within NHD sessions (210 minutes). This format is similar to the operation of outpatient clinics and radiology sessions. The following assessment considers the time element for procedures grouped by complexity.

It would be reasonable to expect a single consultant to complete the following number of procedures/patient episodes:

Diagnostic imaging – *in vitro*, typical case mix per NHD	Patients (no.)
Routine *in vitro* studies or planar images (10 min)	21
Complex tomographic images (15 min)	14
Co-registration studies (30 min)	7
Positron emission tomography (45 min)	4–5
Mixed	Variable

Separate sessions should be identified for cardiac stress testing. Allow 30 minutes per patient (7 patients per NHD).

Outpatient therapy	Patients (no.)
New patients (45 min)	4–5
Follow-up patients (20 min)	10
Mixed	Variable

Inpatient therapy

One or two patients depending on the complexity of the treatment and whether the administration itself is delegated to other trained professionals. Where work is mixed during an NHD, the clinical component can be apportioned pro rata. It is emphasised that the workload estimates listed relate to uninterrupted clinical activity. Efficiency will suffer if clinical sessions cannot be protected. This is more likely to be an issue in small departments where a single consultant may be less able to delegate routine queries to other staff.

In devising work programmes, consideration should be given to the concept of fixed commitments. These include procedures undertaken on a regular basis such as outpatient clinics, special procedures, teaching, ward rounds etc. Duties such as administrative work, teaching and training would be considered flexible commitments.

APPENDIX 1

Basis for estimating time allocation for nuclear medicine procedures

	Time (min)
▓ Routine planar + *in vitro*	
Planar static whole body bone scan	7
Static renal imaging	5
Dynamic renogram	8
Indirect cystography	5
Thyroid image	8
Gated radionuclide ventriculography	5
Breath tests	5
Red cell mass/plasma volume	5
Glomerular filtration rate measurement	5
Bone densitometry	5
Bone marrow imaging	7
Lung ventilation and perfusion imaging	10
White cell imaging	10
Blood pool/haemorrhage	15

Allow 10 minutes per procedure on the basis that simple reports will be balanced by those requiring review of previous studies, other investigations or clinical notes.

▓ Complex imaging – including correlative studies	
Myocardial perfusion imaging	10–15
Bone tomography	10–15
HMPAO brain tomography	15
MIBG/octreotide + tomography	15
Gallium + tomography	15

Allow 15 minutes on average

▓ Image co-registration studies	30
▓ Positron emission tomography	45
▓ Therapy	
Outpatient: New patient	45
Follow-up	20
Inpatient	Variable depending on degree of delegation to other staff. Allow one hour on day of administration and 15 minutes per day for each subsequent inpatient day.

References

1. World Health Organisation. *The medical uses of ionising radiation and isotopes.* Technical report. Series 492: 972.

2. Royal College of Physicians. Nuclear medicine: provision of a clinical service. Working Party Report. London: RCP,1998.

3. British Nuclear Medicine Society. *Nuclear medicine generic quality guidelines for the provision of radionuclide imaging services.* April 2001 www.bnms.org.uk

4. Intercollegiate Standing Committee on Nuclear Medicine. Manpower Survey (in press).

5. Hoefnagel CA, Clarke SEM, Fischer M *et al.* Survey: Radionuclide therapy practice and facilities in Europe. *Eur J Nucl Med* 1999;**26**:277–282.

6. Wells CP, Burwood RJ, Forbes EK. South Thames Nuclear Medicine Survey 1996–97. *Nucl Med Commun* 1997;**18**:1098–108.

7. Ell PJ. Nuclear medicine. *Postgrad Med J* 1992;**68**:82–105.

8. British Nuclear Medicine Society. *Manpower and training survey* (In press).

9. Intercollegiate Standing Committee on Nuclear Medicine. Position paper on strategy for nuclear medicine and radionuclide imaging in the UK. March 2000.

Palliative medicine

i Introduction: description of the specialty and clinical needs of the patients

Palliative medicine was recognised as a specialty in 1987, when specialist medical training programmes were established. This coincided with the rapid development of specialist palliative care services, which included new links between community, hospice and hospital care and between the NHS and the voluntary sector. Since 1995, the development of cancer services following the publication of the Calman-Hine Report has given further impetus to specialist palliative care integrated with cancer services. In particular, this has led to a rapid and continuing expansion in consultant posts. As a consequence of these continuing developments, many consultants in previously established posts are playing a key role in the strategic development of local services, and those taking up new appointments may be doing so without a fully developed or resourced service infrastructure.

Palliative care is the active total care of patients and their families by a multiprofessional team when the patient's disease is no longer responsive to curative treatment (World Health Organisation, *Technical Series 804*, Geneva 1990). The majority of palliative care in the UK is provided within the clinical setting in which the patient is routinely managed, particularly primary care, rather than by specialist services. However, specialist palliative care services are needed by a significant minority of people whose deaths are anticipated, and may be provided directly by specialist services or indirectly by means of professional advice to those caring for the patient. Referral is usually prompted by the presence of severe uncontrolled symptoms, major difficulties in adjusting to a terminal illness, or the need for inpatient terminal care.

Consultants in palliative medicine work within multiprofessional specialist care teams and services. Traditionally, the vast majority of patients referred for specialist care have had advanced cancer. Although that remains the case for many services, the need for palliative medicine is not diagnosis-specific but is defined by the patient's and family's needs. An increasing proportion of patients with advanced HIV disease or end-stage organ failure is now referred to specialist palliative care services, particularly in acute hospitals. Across the UK there is wide variation in the proportion of people dying from cancer who are seen by specialist palliative care services. In 1985 the range was 25–60%. Just under 20% of all cancer deaths occur in hospices or specialist palliative care inpatient units. The proportion of patients seen is determined partly by the availability of services, and rises as services expand. Referrals come equally from hospital services and primary care.

ii Organisation

Primary and community care

Palliative care for patients at home is provided by GPs and community nurses, with advice, where appropriate, from a community specialist palliative care team. As cancer networks develop, the role of GPs in the care of cancer patients is becoming better developed and defined. It is expected that improved sharing of clinical information and clearer patient pathways will also further develop the role of GPs in palliative care. The majority of patients would prefer to die at home if there were sufficient support.

Specialist palliative care teams in the community normally consist of clinical nurse specialists, and possibly other non-medical members such as a specialist social worker, with at least part time input from a consultant in palliative medicine. Each team typically covers a geographical area and liaises closely with the GPs and community nurses in that area.

Secondary care

Every acute hospital should have a specialist palliative care team that includes at least a part time consultant in palliative medicine. In addition to advising on the care of individual patients, the consultant's role includes education, particularly for junior hospital doctors; the development of patient pathways and protocols; and participation in the strategic development of palliative care. The consultant may also be a member of a local clinical ethics committee. The consultant will usually hold at least one outpatient clinic a week, possibly in addition to joint clinics with oncologists, and attend tumour site-specific team meetings.

Many consultants work in a hospital-based team in addition to a role in a community team, and may have responsibility for specialist inpatient beds, which often are not on the site of the acute hospital.

Although no consultant should practise single-handed, at present many do, particularly in the hospital setting. It is vital that the consultant has good links with colleagues in the surrounding network, has adequate time for off-site CPD and participates in clinical audit in collaboration with colleagues from surrounding units.

Tertiary care

Many cancer services are organised on a 'hub and spoke' basis across a cancer network. Patient pathways lead patients to be referred to a cancer centre for radiotherapy and specialist medical oncology, while follow-up and chemotherapy are carried out at a more local cancer unit. Specialist palliative care services in general do not follow this model, because they are organised geographically around patients' homes.

Every cancer centre needs at least one consultant in palliative medicine leading the delivery of specialist palliative care for inpatients. But a larger than usual proportion of the consultant's time will be spent liaising with more local consultants in palliative medicine to whom the patients are already known and facilitating seamless care during the patient's transition back to the local services.

Specialist inpatient units

Most specialist inpatient palliative care units are not on acute hospital sites, although a few are integrated into an acute hospital. Inpatient units admit patients with complex needs for symptom control or with major emotional distress or family problems. A substantial proportion of patients will be discharged following a short admission, usually of the order of two weeks or less. Patients are also admitted for inpatient terminal care if adequate support for a death at home cannot be provided.

The consultant in charge of a specialist inpatient unit will be supported by other medical staff, who may include non-consultant career grades, clinical assistants and possibly an SHO, an SpR or both.

Medical staff are non-resident on call. There are usually only limited investigative facilities. Therefore patients who need acute management of reversible complications, such as neutropenic sepsis following chemotherapy, should not in general be admitted.

iii   Patterns of referral

All referrals to palliative medicine are made after the diagnosis of advanced, progressive and incurable disease has been made. Referrals often follow a long period in which the disease has been managed in secondary care. Referrals may be:

■ Directly from the general practitioner when the terminal nature of the disease becomes apparent, or symptoms are difficult to control

■ Directly from a consultant in secondary care

■ From another specialist palliative care team in another setting or location

■ As a result of an enquiry by the patient or family.

Most services operate within working hours only. Urgent referrals are normally seen within one working day. Admissions to specialist palliative care units can rarely be arranged out of working hours, although an exception may be made for patients already known to the service or who have been recognised as at risk of requiring emergency admission.

Most services offer a 24-hour telephone advisory service to colleagues both in the community and in hospital. They may also provide specialist equipment, such as syringe drivers, for patients at home.

Most referrals are for advice and support. Consultants in palliative medicine typically offer shared care with the general practitioner in the community and with the referring specialist in a hospital setting.

iv   Ways of working, clinical networks and community arrangements

Supportive and palliative care networks

Services for cancer patients are now organised in clinical networks. Palliative care services form part of supportive and palliative care networks, which are subunits of cancer networks, although arrangements differ across the country to recognise local structures and meet local needs. The degree of integration within local cancer services is variable, but in general is increasing.

The majority of inpatient specialist palliative care beds are funded by the voluntary sector and are located in free standing hospices. However, consultant posts are often shared with local DGHs or with trusts providing cancer services. NHS specialist palliative care units may be co-located with acute services. Consultant posts are often so structured that there is palliative medicine input to cancer services in cancer centres, in cancer units within DGHs and within the community, in addition to responsibility for inpatient beds. Consultants in palliative medicine often carry out joint clinics with oncologists, as well as attending tumour site-specific meetings.

Despite the close working arrangements with cancer services, since palliative care is not diagnosis dependent, palliative care networks also liaise with specialties other than oncology.

Community arrangements

Within the community, patients receive palliative care from their GPs. The role of the community palliative care team is advisory. Local arrangements vary, but in some areas GPs with particular interest and expertise in palliative care have taken up posts as facilitators, to promote training in palliative care among local GPs, or as leads locally. Many specialist palliative care units employ GPs as clinical assistants, or have SHOs drawn from the Vocational Training Scheme. This helps to develop considerable expertise in GPs who have held these posts and raises the local standard of palliative care within primary care.

v   Characteristics and features of a high quality service

Since their inception, specialist palliative care services have aimed to provide a very high quality of care, often using charitable funds to provide higher staffing levels and a better care environment than is usual within the NHS. More recently, services have been commissioned to a specification that usually included quality standards. Such standards may be agreed regionally or nationally, and are often verified by a peer review process or external accreditation.

Characteristics of a high quality service include:

- The multiprofessional team includes at least core specialists in palliative medicine, specialist nursing and social work
- At least the lead person in each professional within the team should be a trained and acknowledged specialist in palliative care
- In addition to the core specialties, patients have access as appropriate to other disciplines so that they receive physical, psychological, social and spiritual support
- Management is evidence based wherever possible
- Clinical audit and research programmes exist to evaluate treatments and outcomes
- The service plays a recognised role in both external and in-service education provision, and the education is offered both to professionals wishing to incorporate the palliative care approach into their practice and to those training in palliative care
- Patients and families are involved in management plans and encouraged to express their preference about where they wish to be cared for and where they wish to die
- Carers and families are supported through the illness into bereavement and the needs of the bereaved are recognised and addressed.

(Specialist Palliative Care: A Statement of Definitions. *National Council for Hospice and Specialist Palliative Care Services 1995*)[1]

The *features of* a high quality palliative care service are as follows:

Referral

- Means of receiving referrals rapidly, eg by fax and/or electronic transmission
- Dedicated administrative staff
- Explicit standards specifying the interval from referral to first assessment for urgent and routine referrals.

Medical assessment

- Although not all new patients will be seen by the consultant in palliative medicine, early medical review must be available
- Sufficient time for thorough medical assessment of a new patient, either in the outpatient clinic or on a domiciliary visit. At least an hour is normally required
- Access to medical notes and results of investigations carried out at other hospitals
- 24-hour medical advice available to colleagues in community and hospital settings
- Support from suitably trained nurses
- Dedicated administrative support
- Rapid links to other medical disciplines, particularly clinical oncology and pain anaesthesia.

Day care

- Dedicated day care space
- Trained and experienced nursing support
- A separate clinical room in which medical assessment can be carried out
- Facilities for minor procedures such as blood transfusion, interventional analgesia.

Inpatient care

- Dedicated inpatient beds
- High nurse-to-patient ratio
- Trained nurses with specialist skills and experience in palliative care
- Dedicated social work support
- Spiritual support
- Access to other relevant professionals, eg pharmacist, lymphoedema specialist, physiotherapist, occupational therapist, clinical psychologist
- Dedicated administrative support
- Other forms of support for staff, patients and families, such as complementary therapies, volunteers
- Families able to stay overnight.

Education facilities

- Dedicated teaching space
- Audio-visual equipment
- Educational resources, eg journals, books, videos, access to computerised databases
- Staff with educational experience and relevant qualifications.

Patient information

- Information for patients and families in written form, videos etc
- Information regarding medication regimens.

Links with colleagues

- Arrangements for communicating rapidly with the patient's general practitioner and community nurse when the patient is discharged or dies
- Collaboration with colleagues in the community and in acute hospitals to support patients as their care moves between care environments.

vi   Outline of clinical work of consultants in palliative medicine

Consultants in palliative medicine support the work of specialist palliative care services. Many are still the only consultant in their service. Although the number of trainees has increased, the ratio of consultant to trainee and other medical staff remains high. Palliative medicine is often a consultant-delivered, as well as a consultant-led specialty. A substantial proportion of specialist inpatient services are funded by the voluntary sector, and more than half of consultants in palliative medicine have some or all of their sessions funded outside the NHS.

Consultants support a range of specialist palliative care services including inpatient units, day care, community and hospital support teams. A detailed workload study carried out in 1997 indicated that one whole time consultant would, on average, be responsible for 11 inpatient beds with 220 admissions per year, a home care service seeing 235 new referrals annually, a day hospice seeing 70 new referrals annually and a hospital support team. Support teams both in the community and in hospital are often nurse led, with the consultant seeing only a proportion of the new patients referred, although some consultants see all new referrals personally. There is therefore a wide variation in the proportion of time spent directly seeing patients, the proportion spent supporting and advising other members of the team and the time devoted to teaching, management and the strategic development of services in the area. On average, a consultant is likely to carry out at least two ward rounds per week, and devote 2–3 sessions to seeing outpatients, ward referrals or patients at home. Multiprofessional team meetings are key to team management of patients in palliative care, and consultants are likely to attend 1–2 per week. Increasingly, with the development of site-specific cancer services involving meetings of all the consultants involved, consultants in palliative medicine are also being called upon to attend weekly or fortnightly meetings to discuss patients with lung, breast and other common cancers. Assessment of a new patient is time-consuming, involving often multiple physical symptoms, considerable emotional distress and complex family dynamics. Outpatient sessions therefore allow up to an hour per new referral. Most consultants see 1–2 new patients and up to six follow-ups in an outpatient clinic.

Many consultants work on more than one site. In addition, most provide both outpatient clinics and a domiciliary visit service. Considerable time is therefore spent travelling, and liaising with general practitioners, hospital colleagues and other palliative care services. There is no participation in acute medical on-take work. Nevertheless, because many consultants work single handed, those with responsibility for inpatients, or for 24-hour care in the community, may have an onerous on-call responsibility which may be seven days a week. Some also carry out non-resident first on-call duties.

vii   Work of the other members of the multidisciplinary team

Clinical nurse specialist in palliative care

Nurses with advanced qualifications and experience in palliative care are key members of teams supporting the care of palliative care patients in non-specialist settings.

▌ Community clinical nurse specialists (CNSs) are the largest professional group in community support teams. They assess the physical, psychological and social needs of patients at home, advise GPs and community nurses on the management of symptoms and help to plan future management at home.

▌ Hospital CNSs are also the largest group in hospital support teams. Their major role is to assess the needs of patients, advise on the management of symptoms and play a role in planning for hospital discharge, whether to the patient's home, to a nursing home or to specialist inpatient palliative care.

▌ Some hospital based CNSs work in a site-specific team, dealing with only one type of primary cancer. They see patients with that cancer at different stages, including at diagnosis, and may provide advice and support during primary management as well as when the disease is advanced.

▌ Specialist nurses based in a hospital or a specialist inpatient unit carry out a liaison role, helping to make the transition from the inpatient setting to the community as seamless as possible.

▌ Nurses with a subspecialty training, eg in the management of lymphoedema, run clinics for patients with that problem.

▌ Although rarely trained counsellors, many CNSs provide considerable emotional and psychological support to patients and families.

▌ Community CNSs continue to provide emotional support to families in bereavement, and refer on to specialist services individuals in whom bereavement is causing severe problems.

▌ Some community services provide a 24-hour on-call or crisis response team, of which CNSs are a part.

Specialist social worker

Most inpatient services, and an increasing proportion of other services, include at least one specialist social worker. The roles of such a worker include

▌ Counselling and psychological support to patients and families, including children

▌ Advice on financial problems, including charitable grants and benefits

▌ Liaising with local authority social services in planning care after discharge

▌ Bereavement support, including complex and difficult bereavement problems

▌ Support for other staff within the specialist palliative care service.

Chaplain

Many patients and families seek spiritual help and support as death approaches, including those whose religion is non-Christian or who have no formal religious faith. The chaplain's role is increasingly to offer support tailored to the needs of the individual, to encourage religious leaders from other faiths to visit patients and to give comfort to patients facing death who do not have any religious affiliation.

Therapists and others

An increasing number of services include physiotherapists, occupational therapists, pharmacists, clinical psychologists and a variety of complementary therapists in their teams. They may work with individual patients, or provide group therapy, often in a day care setting. Physiotherapists and occupational therapists are important in the rehabilitation of patients with disability from advanced disease.

viii Conjoined services

- Multiprofessional specialist palliative care team members
- Clinical oncology
- Medical oncology
- Primary care
- Community services
- Respiratory medicine
- Gynaecological oncology
- Gastroenterology and gastro-intestinal surgery
- Voluntary bereavement services
- Major charities offering patient care, eg Marie Curie Cancer Care
- Social services in the community
- Nursing homes.

ix Specialised facilities

In every setting, consultants in palliative medicine and their supporting medical and non-medical teams must be provided with adequate office space, and computer and administrative support.

In acute hospitals

Outpatient facilities should allow:

- The patient and any relevant family members to be seen together, if appropriate
- The consultant to be accompanied by at least one other member of the multiprofessional team
- An unhurried and entirely private consultation to be carried out
- Space for the patient and/or family members to talk separately with a clinical nurse specialist, social worker or other team member
- Specialist drugs to be dispensed promptly, so that long waits are avoided for very sick patients
- Comfortable seating for patients to wait, eg for transport or drugs.

Inpatient wards:

- There should be provision for private conversations with patients and with families, together or separately
- Each hospital should make policy decisions on whether the role of the consultant in palliative medicine is purely advisory, whether care is shared (ie the consultant in palliative medicine can prescribe for inpatients), or whether the consultant in palliative medicine has admitting rights to hospital beds.

In specialist palliative care units

Facilities should wherever possible be integrated. The physical proximity of inpatient, outpatient and day care facilities promotes good communication and the efficient use of consultant expertise and time. If the community team base can be co-located, this further improves communication and allows the community clinical nurse specialists more easily to keep links with their patients during admissions. It is very important that patients and families can access specialist units easily. Therefore where a service covers a wide geographical area it may be more appropriate that there are outlying day care units, or even that the inpatient beds are distributed across one or more community hospitals in addition to a hospice or NHS specialist palliative care unit.

The inpatient unit should provide:

- an adequate number of single rooms, if possible with en suite facilities
- a comfortable, homely environment rather than a clinical hospital-type one
- appropriate equipment for the care of weak, cachexic, debilitated patients, eg pressure-relieving mattresses, electrically operated beds and chairs, easily operated nurse call systems, individual telephones, TVs etc, assisted baths and showers
- comfortable sitting rooms for the use of patients and visitors
- self-catering facilities, so that people can make hot drinks and simple snacks
- private rooms for interviews, counselling sessions etc.
- dedicated space for viewing the deceased relative
- a chapel or spiritual room in which patients and families can pray, meditate or follow the rituals of their religion
- facilities for families to stay overnight.

The day care centre should provide:

- a comfortable environment for people to meet socially
- facilities for a shared meal
- opportunities for therapy, eg art or music therapy, and diversion
- at least one outpatient room in which patients can be medically assessed and nursing procedures performed
- an assisted bath and facilities for washing and setting hair
- appropriate space for complementary therapies such as massage.

In addition, because education is a major function for specialist palliative care, the specialist unit should provide space for teaching sessions and educational resources for the use both of the unit staff and students attending courses.

x   Quality standards

These are, or will be, defined by

- EL(96)85 *A Policy Framework for Commissioning Cancer Services: Palliative Care Services*[2]
- *The National Cancer Plan*[3] and the specific actions identified at regional and network level in both the *NHS Cancer Plan* and the subsequent *NHS Plan – Implementation Programme*[4]
- *The Manual of Cancer Standards*[5] and the specific sections on standards in palliative care expected to be published in 2001[6]
- The Guidance on Supportive Care to be developed by the National Institute for Clinical Excellence (NICE), to be published in 2001[7]
- The Department of Health's Supportive Care Strategy, to be published in 2001.[8]

In addition, standards have been defined in several national or regional accreditation or peer review schemes.

xi Contribution to acute medicine

Consultants and SpRs in palliative medicine do not participate in the on-call rota for acute general medicine. Hospital support teams offer a consultation service for acute problems in palliative and terminal care during their normal working hours; out of hours, telephone consultation from a specialist inpatient service is usually available.

xii Academic palliative medicine

There are few academic departments of palliative medicine, but increasing numbers of SpRs are doing higher degrees during or after their clinical training. The patient population is characterised by a short prognosis, an unstable clinical state, the need for polypharmacy and increasing cognitive impairment as death approaches. Conventional randomised controlled trials are therefore difficult to carry out. Nevertheless, active research both into methods of symptom control and into the cost-effectiveness of models of service delivery is being carried out. Academic departments also make a major contribution to the delivery of clinical services.

xiii Developments offering improved patient care

- *Joint clinics* between oncologists or physicians and consultants in palliative medicine, so that patients receive truly integrated management
- *Palliative care services offering extended hours*, in some cases 24-hour services, to deal with crises
- *Hospice at home* services providing an enhanced level of medical and nursing care for patients at home
- *Link nurse* schemes, offering additional training to one member of each ward or community nursing team so that they in turn can be resources for their colleagues
- *Lymphoedema clinics* have improved the management of chronic lymphoedema, particularly following anti-cancer treatment.

WORK OF CONSULTANTS IN PALLIATIVE MEDICINE

1 Direct patient care

A Work in the specialty

Inpatient work

- Ward rounds in a specialist inpatient unit: at least two per week, of which one is a multiprofessional team meeting
- Teaching SpRs and other staff is a significant component of ward rounds
- One WTE consultant is responsible for a median of 11 inpatient beds, admitting a median of 220 patients a year, of whom 188 will be newly referred

▓ Referral work in acute hospitals: a consultant will on average see 200–300 new referrals each year; the range is wide

▓ Full-time consultants spend a median of 4.5 hours per week in indirect clinical care, including supervising specialist nurses, liaison with colleagues and case conferences.

Outpatient clinics

▓ Most consultants carry out one outpatient clinic per week

▓ They see 1–2 new patients and up to 6 follow-ups at each clinic

▓ If a trainee takes part in the clinic, s/he rarely sees more than 1–2 new patients

▓ Clinics may be held at an acute hospital, a palliative day care unit or attached to a specialist inpatient unit

▓ Most consultants work flexibly, and will see urgent referrals on any day of the week either as an outpatient or at home

▓ Consultants working in cancer centres or cancer units will carry out one or more joint clinics with oncologists per week.

Specialised clinics

▓ Some consultants hold clinics for patients with pain problems, including non-malignant pain

▓ Interventional procedures for pain control may be carried out.

Home care

▓ Consultants on average make 1–2 domiciliary visits a week; the range is wide

▓ The median number of referrals for patients at home is 235 per year; the range is wide

▓ The service model varies; some consultants see all new referrals, in other services the majority are initially assessed by clinical nurse specialists

▓ Typically one session each week is spent supervising clinical nurse specialists in the community team.

On-call commitment

▓ The on-call commitment is onerous

▓ Many consultants are first on-call for specialist inpatient beds at least 1:4

▓ Many consultants work single-handed, and have second on call rotas of 1:1

▓ Sleep is rarely disturbed, but the workload for the first on call consultant during a weekend is significant. Time off in lieu is rarely included in job plans.

B Acute medicine

▓ Consultants in palliative medicine do not participate in the on-take rota for unselected medical emergencies.

C Academic medicine

▓ Consultants with academic posts typically make a significant contribution to patient care

▓ They usually participate in hospital assessments and sometimes in specialist inpatient care, including on call rosters.

2 Work to maintain and improve the quality of care

This work encompasses duties in clinical governance, professional self-regulation, continuing professional development, education and training of others. For many consultants, at various times in their careers, it may include research, serving in management, and providing advice. All require consultant participation. Such work is described fully in Part 1 of this document. Its scope is summarised in the Appendix 1 to Part 2. Management and advisory work are identified specifically in the Appendix.

WORKFORCE REQUIREMENTS FOR PALLIATIVE MEDICINE

A detailed survey of the workload of consultants in palliative medicine was carried out in 1997. At that time, 47% of consultant posts were single-handed, and the median ratio of whole-time consultants to non-consultant medical staff (training and non-training) was 2:1. Although trainee numbers are increasing, palliative medicine is predominantly a consultant-delivered service.

The majority of consultants have clinical responsibilities in more than one care setting. In 1997, 88% of consultants had responsibility for specialist inpatient beds, with a median of 11 beds per consultant. The proportion of time spent in clinical work, both direct patient care and supporting other professionals in the team, was highest for part-time consultants but was more than 50% of the working week even for whole time consultants. Non-clinical work, particularly teaching and involvement in the strategic development of palliative care services, took up on average 39% of consultants' time. Few consultants had adequate time for CPD, audit or research.

In determining the consultant requirements in palliative medicine, a number of factors have to be taken into account:

▯ An ageing population. Cancer is the major diagnosis leading to referral for palliative care. Cancer is predominantly a disease of the elderly. WHO estimates the prevalence of cancer will increase markedly by 2010.

▯ Trends in referral of patients with cancer. Referral rates tend to rise as services become available, and reach 70% of the cancer population in some areas. A 70% referral rate has been used in calculating consultant requirements.

▯ Increasing referral of patients with non-cancer diagnoses. Research indicates that patients with non-malignant terminal illnesses have at least as many problems, in terms of symptoms and social and psychological needs, as those with cancer. In some services that have encouraged referral of patients with non-malignant disease they now account for 50% of referrals. A conservative estimate of 20% has been used.

▯ A high proportion of female doctors in the specialty. Many train part time and a proportion wish to continue in part time work as consultants.

▯ The workloads measured in the 1997 survey were too high to allow adequate time for CPD, audit, research and clinical governance and therefore did not facilitate the delivery of a high quality service.

Based on calculations including all these factors, in England there should be a minimum of 1 WTE consultant in palliative medicine for every 160,000 residents. The National Cancer Plan envisages that the number of consultants in palliative medicine in England should double by 2009. The current number of SpRs in training is adequate for this increase.

Calculation of consultant requirements

RCP baseline 80,000 resident population	218.6 cancer deaths per annum
If 70% access specialist palliative care	153 referrals/year
Add 20% non-cancer referrals	184 referrals/year
Requirement if one WTE sees 360 new patients/year	0.51WTE
Minimum consultant requirement (WTE)	1 per 160,000 residents
Minimum consultant numbers assuming 30% work part time	1 per 120,000 residents

This requirement will increase as
- The incidence of cancer rises in an ageing population
- The implementation of the National Cancer Plan increases the requirement for consultants in cancer centres and units
- The number of academic posts increases: at present there are few

NOTE: *In 1999 there was insufficient information available to allow a more precise estimate of the workforce requirements in this specialty. This recent estimate provides a firmer basis for workforce planning but this too will need to be reviewed in the light of developments in practice and service delivery.*

WORK PROGRAMME OF A CONSULTANT IN PALLIATIVE MEDICINE

Direct patient care

Work in the specialty	Workload	NHDs allocated	Clinical support	Conjoined services
Inpatient work	11 beds; 220 admissions per year	2	Junior medical staff; nursing staff with specialist skills; full multiprofessional team	Investigative facilities; pain anaesthesia; close links with oncologists
Outpatient clinics	1 per week; 1-2 new patients and 6 follow-ups per session	1	Clinical nurse specialist; nurse with specialist skills	Oncology clinics; interventional analgesia
Home/hospital/ day care	Wide range, depending on the structure of the post	2	Clinical nurse specialists; junior medical staff	Primary care; other members of the multiprofessional team
On-call for specialist advice and emergencies	1:4 first on-call; up to 1:1 second on-call	1	Junior doctors, training and non-training	
Indirect clinical work	Supervising other professionals in the team, particularly clinical nurse specialists, and advising colleagues	1	Junior doctors	Clinical nurse specialists; primary care

NOTE: most consultants in palliative medicine play a greater role in the strategic development of palliative care services locally than is common in other specialties. On average, 39% of the working week of a full time consultant was spent in non-clinical work in 1997, largely because of commitments to teaching, strategic development and management roles.

References

1. *Specialist Palliative Care: A Statement of Definitions.* National Council for Hospice and Specialist Palliative Care Services, 1995

2. *A Policy Framework for Commissioning Cancer Services: Palliative Care Services.* EL(96)85.

3. *The National Cancer Plan.* Department of Health, 2000.

4. *NHS Plan – Implementation Programme.* Department of Health, 2000.

5. *The Manual of Cancer Services Standards.* Department of Health, 2000.

6. Specific sections on standards in palliative care. To be published in 2001.

7. Guidance on Supportive Care. To be developed by the National Institute for Clinical Excellence (NICE) (To be published in 2002).

8. *Supportive Care Strategy.* Department of Health. To be published in 2001.

Rehabilitation medicine

i   Description of the specialty

Rehabilitation medicine assists people with disabilities to achieve and maintain optimal physical, mental and social function. It seeks to empower the disabled person, and reduce the impact of disabling and handicapping conditions. This requires established medical skills, provision of assistive technology and environmental adaptations, and the ability to influence social attitudes.

Rehabilitation medicine can be delivered only by an integrated inter-disciplinary team, of which the consultant in rehabilitation medicine is a member.

Disability may stem from congenital or acquired conditions. Disability in children and disability in elderly people are largely covered by the specialties of paediatrics and geriatrics respectively. Rehabilitation medicine has developed as a specialty primarily to meet the needs of disabled people during the intervening period of adult life (often referred to as the sixteen to sixty-five age group). Although the basic principles and individual techniques used are not age-specific, there is good evidence that adults with disabilities require different programmes from those required by elderly people. Nonetheless, there are areas of rehabilitation, particularly relating to technical aids, where services cover people of all ages; for example, the provision of wheelchairs, orthotics and prosthetics.

Rehabilitation medicine covers a considerable number of disabling conditions. Most arise from neurological conditions such as traumatic brain injury, stroke, multiple sclerosis, Parkinson's disease and motor neurone disease. There are greater numbers of people with musculo-skeletal disabilities but only a relatively small number require the specialist skills of Rehabilitation medicine. Conditions arising in childhood such as cerebral palsy, spina bifida, myopathies and dystrophies carry over into adult life and patients need continuing support, advice and assistance. Amputation or congenital limb reduction deformity require life long technical assistance. Other technological provision such as environmental control units, and prescription of wheelchairs, prostheses and orthoses are not disease specific and cover a vast range of disabilities.

The type of disability also has a bearing on the type of service required. At the onset of an illness people require a more medical model of care. However, for those with static conditions, once maximum functional improvement has been gained, services are really there to assist them. For those with relapsing or unremitting disabilities a more supportive framework is required which attempts to empower the individual to manage their own disability, prevent secondary deformity, and which provides the necessary support and treatment when medical intervention is required.

ii   Organisation of the service

Rehabilitation medicine is a relatively new specialty and even now provision is far from optimal.[1] Until recently specialist rehabilitation has been provided in tertiary units, usually at a supra-district, regional or even supra-regional level. This pattern of organisation has been dictated partly by the need for the inter-disciplinary care teams and occasionally by the complexity of technical assistance required to deliver that care.

Disabled people themselves have been vocal in promoting the more accessible services away from traditional acute services. Community rehabilitation is beginning to develop via outreach services or community based locations. This will allow much better conjoined working with primary care services. More critically it aims to maintain the disabled person within the community, should they wish, whilst providing them with information and support to allow them to manage their own lives.

Historically, services in secondary care have consisted of individual therapy services working in relative isolation. However the evidence for the effectiveness of stroke units[2] has highlighted the importance of coordinated interdisciplinary team working. This is likely to be developed further with intermediate care.

iii   Patterns of referral

In common with many other medical specialties referral to specialist rehabilitation services may come from primary care physicians and consultant colleagues. However, because of the multi-faceted nature of rehabilitation many paramedical colleagues also refer into specialist services; indeed disabled people themselves should be enabled to self-refer where that is appropriate.

iv   Ways of working

Rehabilitation medicine encompasses a wide range of skills and the doctor has an unusual role. It differs from a conventional medical role and may not be well understood by medical and lay colleagues. The hallmark of rehabilitation medicine is working as an integral part of the inter-disciplinary team, often leading from within. This combines leadership with an ability to empower other team members. Indeed the consultant in rehabilitation medicine may find him/herself justifying team decisions that differ from their own!

Ideally, all rehabilitation should be focussed around specific goals, set in conjunction with the patient, their relatives and other carers, and agreed with the team.

Many specialist interdisciplinary teams work on a hub and spoke mechanism and this pattern has been recommended in the recent Audit Commission Report.[3]

v   Characteristics of a high quality service

A high quality rehabilitation medicine service will have a robust interdisciplinary team which works as a cooperative autonomy, each individual respecting and understanding the skills of the others. Such team working needs to be developed and fostered. It particularly needs good listening, communicating and negotiating skills. Information sharing and resolution of conflict within the team members are also essential functions.

A typical rehabilitation medicine team involves a consultant in rehabilitation medicine, rehabilitation nurses, physiotherapists, occupational and speech and language therapists, psychologists, social workers and administrative staff. Other professionals might include prosthetists, orthotists, rehabilitation/clinical engineers, technical support workers, dietitians, art and music therapists and podiatrists.

It is increasingly recognised that a named 'case manager' from within the team improves the quality of communication and co-ordination of the process of care.

vi The clinical work of consultants in the specialty

Irrespective of the particular disabling condition, the consultant in rehabilitation medicine has certain primary duties. They are:

1. To facilitate interdisciplinary care.
2. To identify and achieve rehabilitation goals with the patient, their family/spouse/personal assistant and relevant members of the team.
3. More medical duties including:
   - to ensure that the diagnosis and prognosis are accurate, and that they are understood by the patient and others who need to know to ensure that treatments given for associated conditions preserve optimum function with the least side effects
   - to ensure that the management of medical conditions is integrated with the rehabilitation programme
   - to advise on the medical complications of the disabling condition and to provide effective preventative, ameliorative or remedial treatment.
4. Acting as an advocate to:
   - provide information to support medico-legal proceedings
   - negotiate with funding authorities
   - resolve conflict/disagreement whenever needed.
5. Counselling includes family support for specific issues such as work and sexual functioning.

vii The work of the other members of the multidisciplinary team

Nursing staff Rehabilitation nurses have a crucial role, as they are the only functional staff who are with the patient 24 hours per day. They carry over the skills learnt in therapy into daily tasks. This often involves supervising a task, recognising that this takes longer than doing the task for the patient. Specialist nurses, either disease specific (eg M.S.) or symptom specific (eg continence), are increasingly being developed.

Occupational therapists Occupational therapists work on strategies to promote independent daily living, but if this is not achievable will advise on appropriate aids and adaptations to facilitate this as far as possible. For patients who are unable to walk, a fundamental role is to provide a suitable wheelchair, with appropriate cushioning.

Other specialised activities include training upper limb amputees and survivors of stroke in dexterity and bimanuality and assessing the use of I.T. to support communication and environmental access.

Occupational therapists perform psychiatric tests to assess cognitive function. They also work very closely with their colleagues in social services to facilitate reintegration into the community.

Physiotherapists Physiotherapists work on restoring and maintaining joint range, muscle power and balance to facilitate walking, where appropriate. They use various techniques; for example, handling, positioning and splinting, to normalise tone. Other interventions include pain relief and promoting strength and cardiovascular fitness.

Speech and language therapists Speech and language therapists work on all aspects of communication including language, phonation, articulation and the use of communication aids. They also advise on various aspects of swallowing, including stimulation programmes and graded consistency of diet. They may initiate specialist investigations such as video fluoroscopy. If the patient has a tracheostomy, they may co-ordinate a weaning programme.

Dietitians Dietitians work closely with speech and language therapists to ensure a correct diet is supplied. They are critical in tailoring the calorific intake to the changing metabolic requirements of patients recovering from acute injury.

Clinical psychologists Clinical psychologists assess the psychological impact of disability and they work to ameliorate this through counselling, behavioural management and retraining programmes. They advise on formal psychiatric intervention if it is felt this is required. They also support team members dealing with difficult behavioural problems.

Neuropsychologists have an important role in psychometric testing, evaluating a patient's ability to understand, think and remember, plan ahead and make judgements. This informs therapy intervention to target the problems identified.

Art and music therapists Art and music therapists may be particularly useful when communication is impaired and alternative means of expression need to be explored.

Social workers Social workers will provide information on a variety of issues to assist and empower the individual in returning to the community. They may have a specific role in liaison with Social Services or residential institutions regarding discharge from hospital, and they may be involved in setting up care packages for patients who still have a degree of dependency. Social workers frequently provide counselling support for patients, their families and other carers.

Counsellors Informal counselling may be provided by all members of the interdisciplinary team. However, trained counsellors utilise a variety of techniques to explore problems. Counsellors who have experienced disability themselves may be very valuable.

Prosthetists and orthotists Prosthetists assess artificial limbs or orthotic appliances for manufacture and fit, and orthotists maintain them.

Engineering staff Engineering staff are intimately involved with the design, supply and maintenance of assistive, technological devices; for example, wheelchairs, environmental control units and specialised wheelchair seating. Recent advances in technology have created new requirements for the design of integrated systems.

viii Conjoined services

Rehabilitation medicine has links with all medical and surgical specialties. Examples are:

- Paediatrics and geriatrics: at either end of the age range
- Orthopaedic surgeons: joint surgery, tenotomies, amputations (also vascular surgeons)
- General surgeons and gastro-enterologists: PEGs and 'ostomies'
- ENT surgeons: tracheostomy
- Anaesthetists: pain management and sedation for minor procedures in brain-injured patients

▪ Neurologists: epilepsy management and diagnostic advice

▪ Neurosurgeons: shunts, haematoma evacuation, intrathecal pumps

▪ Psychiatrists: disturbances of mood and behaviour, especially when cognitive problems are present

▪ Urologists: continence management.

Specialist rehabilitation medicine services also need to link in with primary care and community services in common with other medical specialties. However, in terms of reintegration into the community a whole range of support needs to be accessed (or accessible in its widest meaning) depending on age, life-style requirements and degree of disability/handicap. Examples of such services include consumer groups and the voluntary sector, education, employment, engineering, housing, social services.

Lastly, rehabilitation medicine services increasingly need to work with legal services to assist those requiring compensation for acquired disability, to ensure that their resulting compensation includes the appropriate elements and is realistically costed.

ix Specialised facilities

Inpatient unit

For a population of 250,000, meeting the needs of adults in the age range of 16–65 is likely to require 15–20 beds. Fifteen beds is the minimum size that is likely to be viable for an interdisciplinary team.

The beds must be located together in order to provide an appropriate environment for rehabilitation and make best use of the rehabilitation nursing complement. Some accommodation must be available in single rooms, but space must be available to therapy, recreation and social activities, team meetings, case conferences and individual therapy.

The inpatient unit must have immediate access to acute medical services as well as psychiatry, neurology, rheumatology, orthopaedics, urology, dietetics and enteral feeding services. The usual range of pathology and radiological services should be on the same site.

The unit must have a supply of wheelchairs, including electric chairs, immediately available for patients on the unit. There will also need to be access to specialist orthotics, special seating and wheelchair clinics.

Outpatient facilities

Specialist rehabilitation has historically been provided on a tertiary basis. Whilst conventional outpatient facilities may meet the needs of some patients undergoing rehabilitation, the majority need access to the interdisciplinary team. Therefore day assessments, case conferences or outreach visits are often more appropriate.

Whatever the pattern of outpatient services, the consultant will need access to:

▪ Gymnasium and hydrotherapy resources

▪ Light and heavy workshops

▪ Continence and stoma care services

WORK OF CONSULTANTS IN REHABILITATION MEDICINE

1. Direct patient care

A In the specialty

Inpatient work

Inpatient work will vary depending on the type of specialist rehabilitation being provided, but the following is amalgamated from a spectrum of sources.

- *Ward rounds:* a multidisciplinary weekly ward round for 20 beds takes 4–5 hours.
- *Referral work:* 10–12 per week.
- *Interdisciplinary liaison* is the hallmark of rehabilitation medicine and requires considerable communication skills, listening skills and liaison. Allow 1 NHD/wk for interdisciplinary liaison in an inpatient rehabilitation unit. Interspecialty liaison will take considerably greater time as rehabilitation overlaps with almost every other surgical and medical specialty. A great deal of time, probably 2 NHDs/wk, is spent actually negotiating, discussing and planning with other colleagues (medical and non-medical)
- *Case conferences:* two to three per week each lasting one to two hours – allow 1NHD.

Outpatient work

- *Specialty clinics*
- *Conventional outpatient clinics* As previously mentioned, these do not lend themselves readily to the specialty, which is largely tertiary based. Where they are still in use, 2–4 new patients or 2–6 follow-ups may be seen in a session of 1NHD
- *Special clinics within the specialty* These can be done either on the specialised unit or on outreach. Examples include:
  School leavers clinic (in conjunction with paediatrics)
  Prosthetics (specialised unit)
  Specialised wheelchair seating (specialised unit or outreach)
  Electric indoor/outdoor powered chairs (specialised unit or outreach)
  Environmental control service (outreach)
- *Acute general medical clinic* Very few rehabilitation medicine consultants are involved in acute take. Even if they do acute on-call they would tend to refer patients on to their specialist colleagues and only follow up those with chronic disabling conditions.
- *Non-acute general medical clinic* For the above reason there will be few rehabilitation medicine consultants who do non-acute general medical clinics.

Specialised investigative and therapeutic procedure clinics

At present these are mainly concerned with spasticity; for example, Botulinum toxin clinics and Phenol blockade services (local and intrathecal). The use of Botulinum toxin is still developing but clinical guidelines have recently been published.[6] To give some idea of the current uptake, it is estimated that:

75% of patients with severe traumatic brain injury

20% of patients with stroke and

60% with moderate to severe MS

will require specific anti-spasticity treatment.[6]

Other therapeutic procedures, such as splinting, tracheostomy and PEG insertion, are done in conjunction with other specialties or as multidisciplinary clinics.

Specialised services within the specialty

Some have already been alluded to. Assessments for disabled drivers are largely linked to rehabilitation medicine services. Patients with neurological disabilities who require specialised urodynamic and fertility advice will be seen in conjuction with the appropriate specialties.

It is worth mentioning that in tertiary units many rehabilitation medicine physicians have a proactive management role and in effect are clinical directors of their units.

Services outwith the base hospital

Some of these services have been covered under the description of outpatient work. However:

▓ Domiciliary work would entail two to three visits per week.

▓ Hospice work is not a particular feature of rehabilitation medicine at the moment but there is clearly an overlap with palliative care in certain rapidly progressive conditions, particularly when they are painful; a specific example is motor neurone disease. Young people with conditions such as muscular dystrophy are managed within their own homes and with their families, as far as possible.

On-call for specialist advice and emergencies

All consultants running specialist inpatient facilities will need to be part of an on-call rota. The exact burden will depend on the number of consultants involved in the unit and the experience of junior staff. With a unit of 20 beds, whilst a consultant may be on call 1 in 2 or 1 in 3, it is unlikely that they will need to come into the hospital more than once a month.

B In acute medicine

As already indicated, only very few rehabilitation medicine consultants also work in acute medicine. This is purely because the demands of acute medicine tend to dominate available time at the detriment of rehabilitation medicine. During the emergence of the specialty therefore it has been found to be preferable to work in the specialty on its own. It should also be noted that the pace of acute medicine and rehabilitation medicine are so very different that different skills are needed, and the two are not *natural* partners.

C In academic medicine

At the moment, for the reasons already stated, there is no recognised career path in academic rehabilitation medicine. This must be addressed.

2. Work to maintain and improve the quality of care

This work encompasses duties in clinical governance, professional self-regulation, continuing professional development, education and training of others. For many consultants, at various times in their careers, it may include research, serving in management, and providing advice. All require consultant participation. Such work is described fully in Part 1 of this document. Its scope is summarised in Appendix 1. Management and advisory work are identified specifically in the Appendix.

WORKFORCE REQUIREMENTS FOR REHABILITATION MEDICINE

As a general statement, the specialty would wish to see one whole time equivalent consultant physician per 250,000 of the population. However, a survey of rehabilitation medicine medical staffing in 2000[1] showed that not one health region in the UK currently meets this minimum standard.[5]

Rehabilitation medicine is too heterogenous for a list of workforce requirements to be exhaustive. Examples are as follows:

		NHDs
Stroke/traumatic brain Injury/complex disability		
Prevalence: ?50 per 250,000 of the population		
Inpatient work		6
Outpatient work		2
	Total	8
Multiple sclerosis		
Prevalence: 300 per 250,000 of the population		
Inpatient work		2
Outpatient work		5
	Total	7
Spinal cord injury		
Prevalence: 125–150 per 250,000 of the population		
Combined inpatient and outpatient work		1
Amputees*		
Prevalence: 200 per 250,000 of the population		
Outpatient work		1
Special seating*		
Prevalence: needed by 100 per 250,000 of the population		
Outpatient surveillance		0.5
Environmental control service*		
Prevalence: needed by 18 per 250,000 of the population		
Outpatient surveillance		0.25
	Total NHDs/week	**18**

* These are not age-specific and cover birth to death.

Additionally, the services are usually run on a regional basis to ensure sufficient patient numbers to maintain expertise.

NOTE: *In 1999 there was insufficient information available to allow a more precise estimate of the workforce requirements in this specialty. This recent estimate provides a firmer basis for workforce planning but this too will need to be reviewed in the light of developments in practice and service delivery.*

For several reasons the workload of a consultant in rehabilitation medicine is increasing.

1. The prevalence of neurological and musculo-skeletal disability is increasing as people survive previously fatal accidents.

2. Additionally people with long-term neurological disabilities are enjoying increasing longevity, thereby further increasing the prevalence of all of these conditions.

3. Many individuals living with disabilities need assistive technology to empower them. Demand for these services is therefore also increasing year by year.

4. An audit project indicates that GPs currently do not have the knowledge to be able to look after people with complex neurological disability and maintain them in the community. A great deal is being invested in these people's optimum rehabilitation after the illness or injury, but this benefit is not being maintained once they are discharged. There may be a case therefore for rehabilitation physicians becoming more proactive in follow-up in the community with outreach services.

References

1.   British Society of Rehabilitation Medicine. Manpower Survey, April 2000.

2.   Langhorne P, Williams B.O, Gilchrist W, Howie K 'Do stroke units save lives?' *Lancet* 1993;**342**:395–98.

3.   Fully equipped. The provision of equipment to older or disabled people. Audit Commission. March 2000.

4.   Turner-Stokes L, Williams H, Abrahams R, Duckett S. Clinical standards for inpatients specialist rehabilitation services in the UK. *Clin Rehab* 2000;**14**:486–80.

Renal medicine

i   Introduction

Renal medicine, or nephrology, includes the care of patients with all forms of renal disease, with or without impairment of renal function. The exceptions are patients with malignancy of the renal tract and other surgical conditions, who are dealt with by urologists. In addition, nephrologists provide the bulk of care for renal transplant recipients, in both the acute post-operative period and in long-term follow-up. Children with renal disease, usually up to the age of 15 years, are cared for by paediatric nephrologists. In many centres nephrologists provide the hypertension service.

It is accepted that renal replacement therapy should be offered to all patients who are likely to benefit.[1] With removal of age limits, and an increasing Asian population in whom the incidence of renal failure is four times that of the white population, the need for dialysis services has much increased. In the 1970s approximately 20 per million population were accepted for long-term renal replacement therapy. The figure is now over 100 per million and up to 120 per million in some areas. In addition, with new guidelines on target blood pressure in essential hypertension,[2] more patients with hypertension are being referred to hospital clinics.

ii   Organisation of the service

Nephrology is predominantly a secondary care service, with the majority of outpatient referrals coming from general practitioners. There is also a large component of tertiary care with acute referrals from cardiothoracic, vascular and hepatic surgery and from urology. In addition, there are many referrals from general physicians and diabetologists.

Primary care

There is only a limited role for the care of renal patients in primary care. Renal disease is not common and general practitioners do not usually undertake supervision of renal problems. Care can be shared, however, with the GP checking blood pressure and undertaking biochemical monitoring between hospital appointments. This reduces the burden of hospital visits.

Secondary care

The specialist facilities and staffing required to support a renal medicine service can usually only be justified in hospitals that service a large population (but see below). One consultant nephrologist per 117,000 of the population is required to provide an adequate service, because of the very heavy on-call load nephrologists should work ideally in teams of five, to provide an acceptable on-call rota. Therefore there should be one large renal unit for a 600,000 population, ideally with outreach clinics serving smaller hospitals.

Tertiary care

Because renal disease is relatively uncommon, general physicians and surgeons are not familiar with its management, and they usually refer patients to a nephrologist at a very early stage. Patients with acute renal failure should always be referred to a nephrologist, although physicians in intensive therapy often share care. Patients with chronic renal failure are always referred to a nephrologist because the necessary facilities and expertise for their treatment are available only in a renal unit. However, this model is not universally applicable for geographical reasons. It is vital to provide a renal service close to the patient and some smaller units are necessary, eg in Carlisle, Cumbria, where the population is small but remote from the main centres at Newcastle and Manchester. The population served would often not justify five whole time consultant nephrologists and this may be dealt with either by having a mix of full time nephrologists with GIM physicians with an interest in nephrology, or a smaller number of nephrologists but with more per unit population to compensate for fewer junior staff and with more frequent on call work compensated by more days off. The higher consultant staff to patient ratio would make days off possible.

iii Special patterns of referral

Referrals from surgical specialties within a regional or subregional unit, or from a smaller hospital without a renal unit, usually occur when an acute complication has arisen. Increasingly, however, pre-operative referrals are made when complications are foreseen. Protocol referrals come from diabetologists when plasma creatinine exceeds 150 micromol/l.

To determine the urgency of an appointment all referral letters should be seen by a nephrologist. Most referrals need to be seen quite urgently and nephrologists do not usually, therefore, have long waiting lists. In consequence clinics are usually very large.

iv Ways of working

There are different patterns of work. In some units consultants share patients; in others each patient has a designated consultant responsible for care. In both systems the consultants cross cover for on-call, and if geography allows there may be cross cover between hospitals.

There is usually an 'open door' policy for pre-dialysis, dialysis and transplant patients, so that they can self-refer without being first seen by their GP.

Multispecialty clinics

Because they are an extravagant use of scarce consultant nephrology time, there are few multispecialty clinics. However, they are important in:

▪ Obstetrics
▪ Renal transplantation
▪ Diabetic care

v Essential requirements for a high quality renal service

1. Sufficient consultant nephrologists supported by high quality medical secretaries and satisfactory office accommodation and IT. There should be sufficient consultants to allow all patients presenting to the unit to be seen by a consultant within 24 hours, usually after initial assessment by a junior.

2. Sufficient junior staff to provide support for ward work throughout the 24-hour period as well as outpatient clinics (or in their absence a greater number of consultants). The juniors must have ready access to a consultant throughout the 24 hours. They must be supported by a phlebotomist and a ward clerk.

3. Sufficient trained renal nurses to undertake the specialised care on the ward, in the community, in the dialysis unit and in outpatients clinics. A structure must be in place to train these nurses since there is quite a high turnover rate.

4. Nurse practitioners are also necessary to co-ordinate the management of anaemia, arteriovenous fistulae and to run an outpatient clinical investigation area.

5. Renal dietitians.

6. Renal social workers.

7. A strong team of transplant co-ordinators.

8. A computer system with a computer manager to collect and collate data to allow participation in the national Renal Registry and thus allow audit of performance against national standards (ref 3, the document currently being revised).

9. A high quality specialty manager, often with experience as a senior nurse in a dialysis unit. The manager organises nurse training as well as ensuring adequate staffing for all aspects of the units work and purchasing equipment and negotiating contracts.

10. Sufficient places for hospital haemodialysis which should include provision to support the peritoneal dialysis and transplant programmes. There should also be satellite haemodialysis units to provide a service close to the patient's home. To support a take on rate of 100 new patients per annum, avoiding the use of the unpopular night (fourth) shift and to allow patients to select haemodialysis rather than CAPD if they prefer it, then 35 haemodialysis stations are required per million population. If, as predicted, the number of patients requiring dialysis rises to 120 per million population, then at least 50 haemodialysis stations per million population will be required.

11. Sufficient inpatient nephrology beds to cope with patients with acute renal failure, newly presenting chronic renal failure, renal transplant patients with complications and haemodialysis and CAPD patients of whom each on average spend 15 days per annum in hospital. The number of beds required is currently 37 per million population. If, as predicted, the dialysis take-on rate increases to 120 per million, then an increased number of beds will be required.

12. A unit to train patients for home haemodialysis and a separate unit for training for CAPD either in hospital or in the community. These units must be staffed by highly trained nurses.

13. A separate renal transplant unit with 6 beds per million population served.

14. Good laboratory, radiological and medical physics support services with a specialist renal pathologist and availability of urgent reports on renal biopsies.

15. A well organised pharmacy service to supply and monitor the use of new and often toxic drugs, and dialysis solutions.

16. Access to a medical library.

17. Access to the internet.

18. Adequate space in outpatient clinics. Patients with renal disease require follow-up for life in specialised clinics – general renal, vasculitis, low clearance, haemodialysis, CAPD and transplant clinics. The ratio of follow-up to new patients is approximately 12:1. Sufficient space for this must be available. The only specialised equipment required is a good quality microscope for urine microscopy but rooms should be equipped with computer terminals to allow access to laboratory results. These clinics must be open access for all patients with chronic renal disease or renal transplant to allow immediate access. A phlebotomist must be available in every clinic.

vi   Characteristics of a high quality service

A service in which all patients can be seen promptly by an experienced nephrologist and in which all necessary investigations are available when needed, whatever the time of day or week. Support services, including dietitian and social worker, should be readily accessible. Staff should have sufficient time to talk to patients and to attend to their own needs for continuing education.

Outpatient clinics should allow sufficient time for each patient to be thoroughly assessed. Currently a new patient should be allowed 30 minutes and a follow-up 15 minutes, if seen by a consultant working alone. If a junior doctor is assisting and sees patients then 60 minutes should be allowed for each new patient, and 30 minutes for each follow-up patient. This allows for a slower rate of assessment (because of lesser experience) and the time necessary to discuss the patient with the consultant. Thus, a consultant working alone can see seven new patients or 14 follow-up patients in a $3^1/_2$ hour session. A consultant working with a junior doctor can together see either 11 new patients or 21 follow-up patients. Staff grade and associate specialist doctors should be expected to work at the same rate as a consultant.

vii   The clinical work of consultants in the specialty

The main duties of a consultant are listed below:

---

1. Outpatient consultation with patients with any type of renal disease for diagnosis and management. Urgent consultations, often same day, need to be available.

2. They often undertake the investigation and management of patients with hypertension. This is almost exclusively in outpatients.

3. Inpatient management of patients with renal disease of all degrees of severity and also of patients with hypertension. This includes the management of acute renal failure developing in patients in hospital with, for example, liver failure. This work is usually accomplished in two major ward rounds each week with in addition consultations on other wards when requested and discussion of emergencies with the SpR.

4. Inpatient and outpatient management of patients following renal transplantation.

5. Nephrologists receive regular calls from ITU, cardiothoracic unit, liver unit and vascular unit as well as from medical specialties. Some are dealt with initially by a trainee and subsequently by the consultant. Many are seen initially by the consultant. In addition, all nephrologists provide a service to acute general medicine when a patient with renal problems presents.

6. Clinical procedures, in particular renal biopsy (now shared with radiologists) and central venous access (again shared with radiologists and surgeons). Some nephrologists undertake vascular access surgery to construct arteriovenous fistulae but this is now unusual. Adequate time for the nephrologist to undertake these vital procedures should be included in job plans.

7. To organise and run an efficient haemodialysis and CAPD service. In addition, a transplant service with a strong organ retrieval service.

8. Nephrologists run renal clinics at surrounding hospitals. Increasingly, satellite haemodialysis units are being established and the nephrologist will usually visit the unit weekly and be available by telephone for problems. Patients with acute renal failure in other hospitals are usually transferred to the centre but this is not always possible and the nephrologist needs to visit the other hospital.

9. On-call duties for general nephrology and renal transplantation usually as a 1 in 3 to 1 in 5 rota.

---

viii   Multidisciplinary team working

Work of nurses in nephrology:

1.   Inpatient care of nephrology patients. This includes the routine care which any inpatient requires, but in addition haemodialysis and CAPD of patients on the ward either for acute renal failure or on the introduction of treatment for chronic renal failure.

2.   Staffing the regular haemodialysis unit. Here the nurses are responsible for most of the routine care, they insert needles for vascular access or gain access to central venous lines. In addition they monitor blood pressure during dialysis and adjust the rate of ultrafiltration and saline infusion to maintain target fluid status and blood pressure. They also administer erythropoietin after appropriate checks on haemoglobin and blood pressure.

3.   The nurses are the main day-to-day contacts for the patients and are often responsible for picking up social problems which may require help to sort out.

4.   Training patients in the technique of CAPD and being the first point of contact for the patients when they dialyse themselves at home. The nurse is often present at the regular outpatient follow-up of peritoneal dialysis patients.

5.   A nurse functions as an anaemia co-ordinator monitoring haemoglobin and ferritin levels and organising iron infusions and erythropoietin injections according to an agreed protocol.

6.   An 'access nurse' monitors arteriovenous fistula flows to pick up problems at an early stage to allow correction of vascular stenoses and fistula aneurysms.

7.   A team of transplant co-ordinators, usually nurses, is required to liaise with other departments, particularly ITUs, and other hospitals to encourage the donations of organs for transplantation. When these co-ordinators are nurses they also assist the transplant surgeons and donor hospital in the retrieval of the kidneys.

8.   A renal 'clinical investigation unit' usually staffed by two experienced nurses is required to allow frequent outpatient monitoring, eg of recent transplant recipients, and to perform iron infusions, blood transfusions and other minor procedures. They may also be responsible for a 24-hour BP monitoring service for other units and GPs.

9.   Training patients for home haemodialysis and visiting the patients in their homes to sort out problems.

10.   Monitoring standards of patient care, eg adequacy of haemodialysis and peritoneal dialysis, blood pressure control and calcium and phosphate control.

Renal dietitian   Renal patients need advice on low phosphate, low sodium, low potassium and often low animal fat diet. Dialysis patients should be seen by a dietitian approximately once every three months. In addition, some patients with chronic renal failure are undernourished and the dietitian is needed to advise on dietary supplements. The dietitian is also often involved in the assessment of the adequacy of dialysis by measuring solute clearance (urea) using the formula Kt/V. The dietician is an important member of the team managing acute renal failure advising on often quite complex regimes of enteral and parenteral nutrition.

Renal social worker   Renal patients are often unable to work because of a combination of a number of factors. These include the time required to undergo dialysis three times a week, general malaise due to less than ideal correction of uraemia, increased vascular disease, the need for antihypertensive drugs, renal bone disease, and in some patients anaemia resistant to iron and erythropoietin. Together with frequent sexual problems this can lead to marital and economic stresses. The input of a social worker may be vital.

Renal pharmacist Renal patients frequently take complex medication regimes and renal pharmacists have an important role both in risk management and in optimising drug therapy.

Specialty manager This is usually, but not necessarily, a nurse. The manager is the key person on the unit, ensuring an adequate supply of suitably trained nurses and technicians for the renal ward and the dialysis unit. The manager is also responsible for balancing the unit budget, in collaboration with the clinical director, by negotiating with purchasers, suppliers and the hospital administration. The specialty manager is active in quality control and is one of the key people in determining the quality of care that can be given.

Electronics engineers Dialysis machines are becoming increasingly sophisticated and with pressure on dialysis units are becoming more intensively used. Reliability is essential and a team of technicians experienced in their servicing is vital. The same engineers are also responsible for maintaining the quality of the water for dialysis.

Medical secretaries There is a massive outpatient load in nephrology, and these patients require close biochemical monitoring. Medical secretaries have the task of recording the results of investigations and of drawing abnormal results to the attention of the doctor responsible, as well as communicating with the general practitioner. Many investigations, often as an inpatient, have to be organised and the secretary is responsible for liaising between ward, radiology or other departments and patient. During normal working hours the secretary is the main link between patient and doctor.

Every consultant needs a personal secretary but there should be additional secretaries responsible for renal transplants and dialysis patients. These secretaries are the first point of contact for transplant and dialysis patients and keep standardised records of results.

Phlebotomists Many renal inpatients and outpatients require frequent blood sampling, and it is vital to have a good phlebotomy service both on the ward and in the clinics.

ix Complementary services

Radiology There must be immediate access to radiology for ultrasound, standard x-rays, CT and MR imaging. In addition, radiology is increasingly undertaking renal biopsy and insertion of central venous lines, and same day service for this is also required.

Renal pathology A specialised renal pathology service is required for renal biopsy interpretation. This service is also required as an emergency service because treatment often depends on precise renal pathology and in some conditions (eg in Wegener's granulomatosis) it must be given within hours of diagnosis, to preserve renal function. The accurate interpretation of the renal biopsy is also important in less acute situations because prognosis and selection of often potentially toxic treatment depend on it. There must be regular, frequent meetings with the renal pathologist.

Medical physics Isotope renography in the assessment of renal structure and function in hypertension, obstructive uropathy and following renal transplant is vitally important. Isotope scanning of the adrenal and parathyroids is also often important.

Transplant surgery The care of transplant recipients is shared with transplant surgeons especially in the first 6 weeks post-operatively. In addition, transplant surgeons provide the vital vascular access surgery service for dialysis patients and the insertion of peritoneal dialysis catheters. In renal units not undertaking transplantation this service is provided by a visiting transplant surgeon or by vascular surgeons.

Urology   Collaboration with urologists is necessary in the management of urinary obstruction, haematuria, renal calculi and urinary tract infection.

Intensive care   Many patients with acute renal failure have failure of other systems, particularly the respiratory and cardiovascular systems, and require ITU care. Good support from an ITU and close working relationships with ITU specialists are essential.

Cardiology   There is an increased incidence of vascular disease in chronic renal failure. Myocardial infarction, arrhythmias and angina are common and may limit suitability for transplantation. A good cardiology referral service, with ready access to CCU is therefore vital.

Residential care   With the acceptance of older patients for dialysis, and ageing of the existing dialysis population, there is a growing need for residential care and for rehabilitation following stroke.

x   Specialised facilities required

The specialised facilities required for a high quality nephrology unit are listed below:

1.   A dedicated nephrology ward staffed by trained nephrology nurses. A proportion of the beds should be staffed to the level of a high dependency unit, with facilities for continuous haemofiltration for the management of patients with acute renal failure who do not require ITU.

2.   A hospital based haemodialysis unit. This provides routine regular dialysis for the bulk of patients with chronic renal failure and also provides the core back up for home dialysis (haemo- or peritoneal dialysis) of patients with problems, failing transplants, patients starting on their dialysis career, and holiday dialysis for patients from other parts of the country (v.s. for number of stations needed).

3.   A training unit for patients to be treated by CAPD.

4.   A training unit for patients to be treated by home haemodialysis.

5.   A dedicated transplant unit (six beds per million population served).

6.   An outpatient clinical investigation unit for frequent biochemical monitoring and with the ability to undertake simple tests and treatments.

7.   Ultrasound equipment to permit siting of central venous lines and renal biopsy on the ward.

8.   Satellite haemodialysis units, depending on the geography of the area covered by the unit.

9.   Isolation cubicles for nursing patients who are infected or who may be infected with MRSA or hepatitis B.

10.   A separate dialysis unit for patients infected with hepatitis B.

11.   Dedicated machines within the main dialysis unit for dialysis of patients infected with hepatitis C or HIV. The number of patients requiring such facilities varies very greatly around the country depending on the composition of the population served.

12.   A room equipped as an operating theatre for minor surgery including insertion and removal of central venous lines and peritoneal dialysis catheters and for renal biopsy.

13.   A consulting room on the nephrology ward to allow patients attending as an emergency outside usual clinic times to be seen.

14.   A consulting room on the regular dialysis unit for regular 3-monthly assessments.

xi   **Quality standards and measures of quality**

A Standards Document was published jointly by the Renal Association and the Royal College of Physicians in 1997[3] (revision in preparation). The performance of renal units in relation to these standards is assessed through the Renal Registry. Most renal units now participate in the registry or have plans to join.

The chief factors that influence access to the service are:

- the distance from a specialised nephrology service
- the shortage of consultant nephrologists
- the severe shortage of haemodialysis places in hospital
- the severe shortage of trained nephrology nurses
- the shortage of inpatient nephrology beds.

These deficiencies affect the safety and quality of the service, as well as access.

xii   **Contribution by consultants in nephrology to acute general medicine**

Sixty percent of nephrologists have responsibility for acute GIM takes and on average devote 30% of their time to GIM. All nephrologists provide a service to acute general medicine when a patient with renal problems presents.

xiii   **Contribution by academic physicians to nephrology**

Fifteen percent of nephrologists have academic sessions, varying from 2 to 11 (full time) per week. The usual academic contract allows 5 clinical sessions plus on-call. Physicians with only 2 academic sessions often find themselves undertaking a full clinical job with little time for research. Those with 5 academic sessions or more usually are able to devote most of this to academic work, as they are perceived to be academics with fewer clinics and fewer referrals. Their on-call commitments are usually the same as those of full time clinical nephrologists.

Most academic nephrologists collaborate with non-clinical medical scientists in their research. These scientists may be biochemists, immunologists, geneticists, physiologists, pharmacologists etc and important discoveries have arisen from such collaboration.

xiv   **Developments that offer improved patient care**

Delay in progression of renal failure   Perfect control of blood pressure to target levels of 120/75 – especially if treatment includes an angiotensin converting enzyme inhibitor (ACE-I) (or probably angiotensin receptor blocker, AT-I blocker) – can delay progression of renal failure in type I diabetes, and in patients with proteinuria greater than 3 gm per 24 hours due to other types of glomerular disease. Much more frequent outpatient visits are required to achieve this goal.

Avoidance of hyperphosphataemia   Phosphate retention in dialysis and pre-dialysis patients leads to hyperparathyroidism often requiring surgery. The use of oral calcium carbonate as a phosphate binder to reduce phosphate absorption is often not effective and may lead to hypercalcaemia.

A new non-calcium binder (Sevelamer) is now available, but it is very expensive and its use will initially be limited to patients in whom calcium carbonate has failed.

Treatment of anaemia Approximately 80% of dialysis patients are currently treated with erythropoietin and usually concomitant intravenous iron. This is expensive and time-consuming but very effective. It should now be available to patients with early renal disease to improve quality of life and prognosis, by reducing the likelihood of left ventricular hypertrophy arising as a result of the high cardiac output consequent to anaemia.

Reduction in rejection of transplants New immunosuppressive drugs are becoming available for renal transplant recipients. These are generally more effective, though often more toxic and more expensive than the older drugs. When these drugs have been fully evaluated they should be available for use by nephrologists in patients who do not respond to, or are unsuited for current therapy.

Adolescent dialysis units At the age of 15 or 16 years children are usually transferred to adult dialysis units. Often they are dialysed alongside elderly patients who often have multiple medical problems. It is agreed that there should be dialysis units dedicated for patients aged 15 to 25 years. Such units do not currently exist.

Centre haemodialysis facilities Some units can only cope with the number of patients by running four haemodialysis shifts over 24 hours, including a night shift, or by encouraging patients to accept CAPD even when it may not be ideal. There is a need therefore for a considerable increase in haemodialysis stations in main renal centres and in satellite units close to the patient's home.

WORK OF CONSULTANTS IN NEPHROLOGY

1   Direct patient care

A Work in the specialty

Inpatient work

- Two ward rounds per week with junior staff, a senior nurse and often a dietitian. These rounds are predominantly to supervise clinical care but also include teaching.
- Referrals from units within the hospital – usually need to be seen on the day of referral.
- Proceduress: renal biopsy, central venous line insertion, PD catheter insertion. Often shared with radiologists and surgeons.

Inpatient and outpatient management of patients following renal transplantation

This is usually done on a rota, with daily rounds during the week on-call. The rota varies between 1 week in 3 and 1 in 5.

Outpatient work

- *General renal clinics*

Most consultants spend around five sessions in outpatients each week because there is a shortage of nephrologists. It is recommended that only three sessions should be undertaken. (Clinics in GIM are additional to this.) The ratio of new to follow-up patients is 1 to 12. The ideal number of patients that can be seen in a clinic has been outlined previously. In practice many more need to be seen and currently 80–100 patients may be seen in a follow-up clinic with one consultant and four juniors.

■ *Special clinics within nephrology*

> Haemodialysis
>
> CAPD
>
> Low clearance (pre-dialysis)
>
> Vasculitis
>
> Hypertension
>
> Joint diabetic
>
> Joint obstetric.

All clinics require support staff including specialised nurses, renal dietitian, and phlebotomist.

Specialised services outwith the base hospital

■ Satellite renal clinics at surrounding hospitals.

■ Satellite haemodialysis units. Weekly visit and with availability by telephone for problems.

These duties require an allocation of sessional time.

On-call for specialist advice

This requires an allocation of sessional time.

Other specialised services within the specialty

■ Organise transplant service with a strong organ retrieval service.

■ Organisation and running of haemodialysis and CAPD service.

These require an allocation of sessional time.

B Acute medicine

Sixty percent of nephrologists have responsibility for acute GIM takes and on average devote 30% of their time to GIM.

These duties, with their on-call responsibilities require an allocation of sessional time.

C Academic medicine

The clinical contribution of academics varies widely depending on their contract and other responsibilities (see section xiii above). Most make a major contribution to the running of the nephrology department.

2 Work to maintain and improve the quality of care

This work encompasses duties in clinical governance, professional self-regulation, continuing professional development, education and training of others. For many consultants, at various times in their careers, it may include research, serving in management, and providing advice. All require consultant participation. Such work is described fully in Part 1 of this document. Its scope is summarised in Appendix 1. Management and advisory work are identified specifically in the Appendix.

WORKFORCE REQUIREMENTS FOR NEPHROLOGY

Consultant NHDs required to provide a service to a population of one million

Calculations are based on numbers of new outpatients, follow-up outpatients, haemodialysis and peritoneal dialysis patients, acute admissions and practical procedures required. The calculations are based on the total clinical load of three centres in the UK (South Wales, Leeds and Newcastle) and take into account the time required for each element of the work; a notional 48-hour working week for consultants; an allowance of 1NHD for administration, audit and management, 1NHD for CME/CPD, 1NHD for teaching and clinical research and 1NHD for on-call commitments.

They show that 94 NHDs are required to serve the nephrology needs of a population of one million. This represents 9.4 WTE nephrologists. If trainees are available (27% of workforce) and associate specialists and staff grades are taken into account then this figure can be reduced to 6.1 WTE per million population. However, 75% of nephrologists have an academic commitment (usually 50% of their time); 60% undertake GIM duties (30% of their time); and that 30% of trainees are women (and may be expected to work 90% of full time). Therefore the figure of 6.1 WTE consultant nephrologists per million population signifies a need for 8.5 physicians per million population, or I for 117,000 population.

However, the dialysis population is expected to continue to grow at least until the year 2020 (as a result of longer survival on dialysis, an ageing population, and an increasing Asian population). It is also predicted that there will be more living donor transplants and this will require additional time for assessment and counselling of donors as well as the peri-operative supervision.

In summary, the current need is for 316 WTE consultants in nephrology (442 physicians) compared to the 164 WTE nephrologists currently in post (230 physicians). With the predicted increase in workload, 390 WTE (546 physicians) will be required by 2006, and 439 WTE (615 physicians) by 2010. To achieve these levels a growth of 11.3% per annum in consultant numbers is required over the next 4 years.

NOTE: *In 1999 there was insufficient information available to allow a more precise estimate of the workforce requirements in this specialty. This recent estimate provides a firmer basis for workforce planning but this too will need to be reviewed in the light of developments in practice and service delivery.*

Conclusion

The number of consultant nephrologists in England and Wales is grossly inadequate to deal with the needs of patients. Current numbers are approximately one quarter of those in France and one half of those in Scotland. There is a need to double the number of nephrologists in England and Wales. An expansion rate of 11% per annum is possible with the numbers of trainee nephrologists currently in post. If we wish to achieve the required consultant expansion outlined above of 8.5 physicians undertaking nephrology per million population, then it has been calculated that the number of trainees in nephrology would need to be increased by 100 for each of the next three years before the numbers could again be reduced.

References

1.   The Kidney Alliance. *End stage renal failure – a framework for planning and service delivery.* The Kidney Alliance, 2001.

2.   Hansson L, Zanchetti A *et al.* Hypertension optimal treatment (HOT) randomised trial. *Lancet* 1998;**351**:1755–62.

3.   The Renal Association. *Treatment of adult patients with renal failure. Recommended standards and audit measures.* Second edition. London: Renal Association and Royal College of Physicians, 1997.

Respiratory medicine

i   Introduction: a brief description of the specialty and clinical needs of patients

Respiratory medicine is concerned with diagnosis, treatment and continuing care of patients with a considerable and challenging range of pathologies. They include:

- asthma
- chronic obstructive lung disease
- diffuse interstitial lung disease
- sarcoidosis
- asbestos related conditions including mesothelioma
- cystic fibrosis
- tuberculosis
- management of chronic and acute respiratory failure
- sleep disordered breathing
- pneumonia
- pulmonary disorders in the immunocompromised host
- bronchiectasis
- pulmonary hypertension
- pulmonary haemorrhage
- pulmonary embolism
- allergic lung disorders
- disorders of the pleura (including mesothelioma, pleural effusion and pneumothorax)
- pulmonary manifestations of systemic disease
- genetic and developmental lung disorders
- a major commitment towards lung cancer, being the most common cancer in both males and females in the United Kingdom.

Sub-specialty interests also include:

- lung transplantation
- cystic fibrosis
- HIV/AIDS
- occupational lung disease
- palliative care and intensive care.

In addition, most respiratory physicians have a major commitment to the care of patients admitted as medical emergencies and in-take and post-take ward rounds. With approximately one-third of all acute admissions being respiratory this commitment is unlikely to diminish. The expectation that all patients with respiratory disease have the option of being reviewed during their inpatient stay by a respiratory specialist, represents a considerable increase in workload.

ii   Organisation of the service

Primary care and community respiratory medicine

Some GPs with an expertise in respiratory medicine provide asthma and chronic obstructive pulmonary disease (COPD) clinics within their surgeries. These are often serviced by nurse specialists. Such services should be developed further in collaboration with the local respiratory physicians and integrated with local services in secondary care. An area in particular where this could be done is respiratory rehabilitation.

Secondary care/inpatient service

Respiratory medicine provides a hospital-based service and respiratory physicians have a major commitment to the care of patients admitted as unselected medical emergencies on selected medical take. All DGHs have at least one consultant with a special interest in respiratory medicine and many have two or three. With appropriate inpatient and outpatient facilities and support, respiratory physicians are able to investigate and manage the vast majority of patients with respiratory diseases locally. The College document recommends no more than 20–25 patients at any one time for a consultant and their team. However, there is a considerable seasonal variation in the workload for respiratory medicine and during winter month's respiratory admissions often exceed capacity in hospitals with no more than two chest physicians. This particular recommendation and others, need to be interpreted in the light of available support from doctors in training, and other health care professions. Additional work requiring specific and itemised recognition in job descriptions, includes on-take responsibilities (see below), post-take ward rounds (see below) and inpatient referral work (equivalent to more than 4 hours per week). The prevalence of respiratory diseases and problems with inpatients under the care of other disciplines, both medical and surgical, which require respiratory specialist input, have a significant impact upon workload.

Tertiary care

Patients with certain conditions, for example, cystic fibrosis, are usually managed in regional centres. Surgical and radiotherapy services are usually based in regional or sub-regional centres. Supra-regional centres exist for the investigation of occupational lung disease, the management of patients with pulmonary hypertension and patients requiring assisted ventilation and the assessment and management of patients requiring lung transplantation.

The future

The BTS is working to achieve a countrywide network of regional centres co-ordinating and, where appropriate, providing specialist care. Each centre should provide access to specialist services for thoracic surgery, sleep related respiratory disorders, ventilatory support, cystic fibrosis, pulmonary hypertension and lung transplantation. These centres would be ideally placed to provide specialist advice on other rare respiratory disease and co-ordinate national programmes of research.

iii Special patterns of referral

Most patients requiring admission are referred by their general practitioner or via the A & E department. Most outpatient referrals are from general practitioners, specialist colleagues in the hospital and the A & E department. Suspected cases of lung cancer need to be seen within two weeks (DH Cancer Initiative). Facilities and resources need to be in place to enable all urgent referrals to be seen promptly. Patients with other life-threatening conditions, such as severe asthma, may need to be seen even more urgently.

iv Ways of working, clinical networks and community arrangements

Respiratory medicine specialists work as members of a multidisciplinary team. The team including career grade and doctors in training, ward-based and outpatient nurses, respiratory nurse specialists, physiotherapists, secretaries and respiratory lab technicians. They liaise with many other specialities, including histopathology, radiology, thoracic surgery and oncology. Clinical networks are being established for lung cancer management and others may follow. There are already strong links between secondary care and primary care with respect to lung cancer care, TB care and asthma care and other links are likely to develop with early discharge of patients with COPD, pulmonary rehabilitation and smoking cessation clinics. Respiratory medicine specialists also work as members of a multidisciplinary team in palliative care, and are also responsible for some HIV work.

v Requirements for a high quality service

A high quality service implies that inpatients and outpatients should receive prompt, expert, effective and compassionate care, and with few exceptions the care they need should be available locally. This requires a well-motivated team that is well staffed and that has access to suitable facilities. In respiratory medicine, respiratory nurse specialists have a very important role. Respiratory specialists should not work in isolation and must have appropriate support staff, including specialist team nurses.

The features of a high quality service are as follows:

Referral:

▮ The availability of 24-hour cover and advice from a respiratory physician
▮ Review of referral letters by respiratory physician
▮ Dedicated support staff
▮ Explicit standards concerning reasonable time from referral to first appointment for urgent and non-urgent patients.

Outpatient clinics:
▮ Dedicated outpatient area
▮ Flexible appointments system
▮ Experienced respiratory nurse specialists to assist in clinic
▮ Pharmacy service available to meet needs identified in clinic
▮ Adequate secretarial staff
▮ Fully supportive Pulmonary Function Laboratory

continued

New patients

▊ General and specialist work: 6 patients per clinic (2 new patients per hour per consultant).

Follow-up clinic

▊ General work: 5 patients per hour, less if juniors are working alongside.

▊ Specialist work: 3–4 patients per. Examples are: review of cystic fibrosis treatment, complex ventilatory problems, and brittle asthma. Trained assistants such as Calman trainees in their last two years, associate specialists, or experienced staff grades, see slightly fewer patients. Junior Calman trainees or SHO's should see half these numbers or less.

Diagnostic services:

▊ *Bronchoscopy:* A maximum of 6 cases per session assuming 2 bronchoscopies per hour: fewer, say 4, if complex procedures are added, or junior doctors are being trained.

▊ Although one session per week is appropriate for most DGH physicians, the incidence of lung cancer varies by 50% between different parts of the country. In high incidence areas, we recommend the allocation of 2 sessions per week to cope with the workload and to comply with the British Thoracic Society recommendations for lung cancer management. 1–2 sessions per week.

▊ Additional sessional requirements are needed if there is a regular commitment to therapeutic procedures such as brachytherapy (3 patients per session) or endobronchial stenting (see below).

Other services:

▊ *Lung cancer.* Although one session per week is appropriate for most DGH physicians, the incidence of lung cancer varies by 50% between different parts of the country. In high incidence areas, we recommend the allocation of 2 sessions per week to cope with the workload and to comply with the British Thoracic Society recommendations for lung cancer management. 1–2 sessions per week. The lead lung cancer physician should be allowed an additional 0.5 session per week to co-ordinate services. If a chemotherapy service is provided by the physician, another 0.5 session per week should be allocated.

▊ *Multidisciplinary lung cancer meeting:* typically should be allocated 0.5 session per week.

▊ *Smoking cessation session* (if provided) would also require typically 0.5 session per week.

▊ *GP chest x-ray service* (if provided) should typically take up 1 session per week.

▊ *Diagnostic sleep services:* Typically 0.5–1 session per week.

▊ *Pulmonary TB – contact tracing:* Typically 0.5 sessions per week. 1 session per week for those seeing more than 100 cases of pulmonary TB per year, or in areas where multi-drug resistant TB is present.

▊ *Occupational lung disease:* Typically 0.5 sessions per month. In specialist referral centres this would be 1–2 sessions per week.

Therapeutic services

Many consultants offer therapeutic services in addition to their routine respiratory work, and job descriptions should recognise them. Not all these services, however, at the present can be achieved. Some areas of work will not need to be done by a consultant, and it is possible, in areas where there is a demand for services, this can be supplied by nurse specialists. Therefore, in certain areas, consultant sessions could be less. Examples are:

▊ *Organisation and provision of long-term oxygen therapy* and other domiciliary oxygen treatment. Comprises laboratory and outpatient work. Typically 1 session per month.

▊ *Treatment of sleep disorders (especially CPAP):* Utilises laboratory facilities. Typically 1–2 sessions per month, in addition to dedicated clinics.

▊ *Respiratory rehabilitation service:* Comprises the organisation of programmes, patient assessment and participation and utilises outpatient and day care facilities. If this service is provided, typically 0.5 consultant sessions per week, though specialist nurse input would need to be considerably greater perhaps 3–5 sessions per week.

continued over

▌ *Treatment of neuromuscular disorders (assisted ventilation):* Utilises laboratory and in-patient services. Typically 2 sessions per month. In specialist referral centres would be 0.5–1 session per week.

▌ *Terminal care:* Many units incorporate terminal care beds with a specified commitment for the respiratory physician. This is in addition to routine workload. Typically 0.5 sessions per week.

▌ *Nebuliser services and asthma support services.* Utilise laboratory and outpatient facilities. Typically 0.5 sessions per week.

▌ *Non-invasive ventilation/acute respiratory failure:* Non-invasive ventilation is rapidly being established as a routine service in most if not all hospitals. The impact on respiratory consultant workload is potentially enormous. The ultimate structure for the service provision is not yet entirely determined. In larger centres this could be in the form of a respiratory HDU, with perhaps 5 sessions per week for the consultant in charge. In many centres this has been established as a ward based, nurse or physiotherapist led service. Consultant supervision however would still account for 2.5 sessions per week in winter months, less in summer.

vi Outline of the clinical work of consultants in respiratory medicine

In addition to their responsibilities for the investigation and management of inpatients and outpatients with respiratory diseases, most respiratory physicians also have a significant commitment to acute general medicine (see details under Direct Patient Care).

vii Outline of the work of other members of the multidisciplinary team

Respiratory nurse specialists make an invaluable contribution to the services that respiratory units are able to offer and the quality of those services. Respiratory nurse specialists undertake many roles, including running asthma clinics, providing education for patients with asthma and liaising with general practitioners and nurses in the community. In many districts the respiratory nurse specialists supervise the domiciliary nebuliser service and assist in the assessment of, and monitoring of, patients requiring long-term domiciliary oxygen. In some units, and this is likely to increase sharply within the next few years, respiratory nurse specialists play the primary role in supervising patients with COPD who are selected for hospital at home care, and for running the pulmonary rehabilitation service. In some units respiratory nurse specialists are employed full time to supervise patients requiring domiciliary non-invasive ventilation (NIV) and continuous positive airway pressure (CPAP) for sleep related breathing disorders. In small units respiratory nurse specialists may undertake many of these tasks together, though increasingly in large units one or more respiratory nurse specialists may be required for each service.

TB liaison health visitors (Nurses) organise and conduct the contact tracing service when patients with TB are identified and they also in many cases supervise that treatment is being taken and chase up patients who default from treatment.

Lung cancer nurse specialists provide an invaluable service counselling patients and their relatives when a diagnosis of lung cancer is made, and advising patients and other health care workers generally on the management of symptoms caused by lung cancer. In some cases they will visit patients at home and in others liaise with other nurses who provide the domiciliary service.

Respiratory function technicians undertake lung function testing of various levels of complexity. In some units they are involved in the sleep service and in exercise testing. Physiotherapists play a very important role in the management of patients with respiratory diseases both for inpatients and outpatients. They also teach patients with cystic fibrosis and bronchiectasis how to undertake postural drainage and help patients with hyperventilation to control their breathing.

viii Conjoined services

The respiratory medicine team has particularly close links with radiology and histopathology in the hospital, and with the local thoracic surgical and oncology units. Close links are also maintained with local palliative medicine services, radiology, histopathology, social services, palliative care, oncology, and thoracic surgery.

ix Other specialised facilities required

Inpatients

▊ Each DGH should have a fully staffed High Dependency Unit/Acute Lung Unit.

Outpatient unit

▊ Sufficient consultation and examination rooms for clinicians and respiratory nurse specialists.

▊ Dedicated outpatient area with rooms large enough for patient, consultant, medical students or other trainees. Natural lighting and additional lighting. Quiet Room for bereavement counselling. An efficient x-ray department in close proximity to the respiratory services is essential

▊ Bronchoscopy suite

▊ Lung function laboratory

▊ Seminar room for unit meetings and multidisciplinary lung cancer meetings.

x Quality standards and measures of quality

The concept of a quality driven service with standards of care clearly defined in contracts, is a framework in which the quality of respiratory medicine for a community can be improved. The standards should be set in relation to:

▊ Referral system

▊ Outpatient clinics

▊ Thoracic surgery

▊ Outpatient treatment

▊ Inpatient care

▊ Discharge from the respiratory service

▊ Training of medical and nursing staff

▊ The availability of the appropriate facilities and equipment

▊ Administration, information and education for patients

▊ Storage and handling of medical records

The contracting process should include the use of treatment guidelines when constructing local arrangements for referral, for shared-care and for clinical audit criteria, which are necessary for quality control. The outcome measures, which might be used, include quality of life assessments and patient satisfaction questionnaires. Guidelines produced by the British Thoracic Society where appropriate with others, cover all the major conditions.

xi Contribution by consultants in respiratory medicine to acute general medicine

Therefore respiratory physicians have a major commitment to the care of acute medical patients. They also have a major commitment to patients admitted acutely with non-respiratory complaints (see details under Direct Patient Care below).

xii Developments that offer improved patient care

There are many, of which the following are examples:

- *Multidisciplinary clinics and multidisciplinary team meetings:* their introduction is largely dependent on organisational factors.
- *Hospital at home schemes for patients with COPD:* their introduction requires the appointment of respiratory nurse specialists but this is offset by the savings in inpatient costs.
- *Development of pulmonary fehabilitation services:* their introduction requires the appointment of respiratory nurse specialists.
- *Nurse-led outpatient clinics.*
- *Acute lung unit:* assisted ventilation for patients with COPD has been shown not only to reduce length of stay, but also to improve survival.

WORK OF CONSULTANTS IN RESPIRATORY MEDICINE

1. Direct Patient Care

A Work in the specialty

Inpatient work

Most respiratory physicians working in DGHs, and also in teaching hospitals, have a commitment to general medicine in addition to caring for patients with respiratory disease, the commitment varying from hospital to hospital dependent on local practices and staffing levels. Most spend at least 60% of their time on respiratory work, and some undertake respiratory work exclusively.

Consultants usually undertake at least two ward rounds per week (ie two sessions) with the respiratory team. Teaching and training are an important component of the ward rounds. With the development of HDUs and specialist care, it is likely that daily ward rounds of patients will become necessary. This could be shared between the consultants on the unit but it is likely to involve each consultant in an additional 0.5 sessions per week. In addition, they have post-take ward rounds in respect of unselected medical admissions, according to the on-take rota.

Ward referrals are seen on the wards or in outpatient clinics as required.

In general, each consultant team should have no more than 20 to 25 inpatients under their care. But with the current drive for patients to be admitted under the care of appropriate specialists, and with the wide seasonal variation in the admission of patients with respiratory disease, respiratory physicians often have more than this number. This has implications for the appointment of additional respiratory physicians. The inpatient work of the majority of respiratory physicians predominantly involves the investigation and management of patients admitted acutely though includes the investigation and management of patients admitted electively. Many units are able to offer a self-admission policy to patients with conditions such as cystic fibrosis, lung cancer or asthma.

Referral work. Respiratory physicians undertake a considerable amount of referral work for patients under the care of other specialists in the hospital (0.5 to 1 session needs to be set aside for this).

Interspecialty and interdisciplinary liaison. Respiratory physicians caring for patients with lung cancer attend weekly MDT meetings with oncologists, thoracic surgeons, pathologists and radiologists. One to two hours need to be set aside for this. Some consultants have close links with the ITU and attend regular meetings. Consultants offering other specialist services such as transplantation assessment and follow up have close links with thoracic surgeons.

Outpatient work

Respiratory physicians see large numbers of respiratory referrals from general practitioners and consultant colleagues. Most see and follow-up patients with a variety of respiratory conditions, though where there are several consultants in the unit it is possible for specific consultants to take the lead for certain conditions (see below under Specialised Services Within the Speciality for details). Most consultants undertake three outpatient clinics a week though some undertake four or five.

New patients: General and specialist work. 6 patients per clinic (2 new patients per hour per Consultant).

Follow up clinic: General work: 5 patients per hour, less if juniors are working alongside. Specialist work: 3–4 patients per hour.

Speciality clinics. It is difficult to be proscriptive about the number of patients that can be seen by a consultant and his/her team as this depends very much on the nature of the patients being seen and on the number and experience of the team. A consultant working alone in a clinic is often expected to see six new patients or 15 follow-up patients, or a combination of the two. Such numbers are increasingly difficult to justify, and it is difficult to offer a high standard of care to those numbers of patients. Trained assistants such as Calman trainees in their last two years, associate specialists or experienced staff grades should see slightly fewer. Junior Calman trainees or SHOs should see a fraction of these numbers.

The number of new patients and follow-up patients seen with complex respiratory problems could be much less than above.

General medical clinics. Respiratory physicians working in DGHs may see new general medical referrals and most see follow-up general medical patients following discharge from hospital. The numbers seen are as above.

Specialised investigative and therapeutic procedure clinics

Bronchoscopy Most respiratory physicians undertake one bronchoscopy session each week. The number of sessions needed will depend on the demography of the local population. No more than six bronchoscopies can be undertaken in one session, and fewer if complex procedures are added such as transbronchial biopsy or if junior doctors are being trained. Additional sessional requirements are needed if there is a regular commitment to therapeutic procedures such as brachytherapy, endobronchial stenting, laser treatment or electrocautery.

Sleep-related breathing disorders This is a rapidly developing subspecialty. Many units are able to offer a basic overnight oximetry service though do not hold dedicated clinics. Some units now offer a comprehensive sleep service and hold dedicated clinics for patients with sleep-related breathing disorders, both for diagnosis and monitoring of patients receiving CPAP treatment. The provision of a comprehensive sleep service requires the provision of one to two sleep rooms and a funded supply of CPAP machines. Consultants providing a comprehensive sleep service spend at least one session a week on this work.

Domiciliary assisted ventilation service This is provided by specialist centres and the sessional commitment to it varies enormously depending on the number of patients seen. With the introduction of domiciliary non-invasive ventilation for patients with COPD in addition to the use of this therapy for patients with neuromuscular disorders it is likely that the sessional commitment of consultants offering this service will increase significantly.

Occupational lung diseases Relatively few units have consultants who offer a comprehensive occupational lung disease investigation service. Consultants working in such units probably spend at least two to three sessions per week on this work.

Specialised services within the specialty

With the increasing requirement for subspecialty work within the speciality of respiratory medicine the individual consultants cannot possibly encompass all the subspecialties and even where there are several consultants in the unit it is not possible to encompass them all and there will always be a need for regional or supra-regional centres for certain services. Examples of specialist services to be expected locally are given below.

Lung cancer Most respiratory physicians investigate and provide supportive care for patients with lung cancer. This is included in their inpatient and outpatient sessional commitment, though the introduction of multidisciplinary team meetings has added 1–2 hours per week to this. The lead lung cancer physician spends at least 0.5 sessions per week co-ordinating services and if clinicians provide a chemotherapy service 0.5 sessions per week needs to be allowed for this.

Pulmonary rehabilitation service This is a rapidly developing service in which patients are seen one to two times weekly for six to eight weeks for education about their condition, support and a supervised exercise programme. The service is largely provided by respiratory nurse specialists and physiotherapists, though may include dietitians and occupational therapists. The lead clinician probably needs to allocate 0.5 sessions per week for this.

Sleep-related breathing disorders – see above.

Non-invasive ventilation for acute respiratory failure Non-invasive ventilation (NIV) is rapidly being established as a routine service in most hospitals. Although in many units the service is largely provided by trained nursing staff and physiotherapists, consultant supervision of this service is essential. In most hospitals one consultant has taken the lead role in supervision of the service and depending on the number of patients requiring NIV could spend at least two sessions a week on this. In large centres, where NIV is also used to assist with the weaning of patients on ventilators in the ITU more sessions would be required. The rapid and necessary growth in acute lung units and high dependency units to maintain those needing respiratory support outside ITUs, has significantly increased the involvement of respiratory physicians in such units.

Pulmonary TB – contact tracing   In most units the consultants see and manage patients with pulmonary TB, although one consultant needs to take the lead for supervision of the contact tracing service and management of difficult cases such as multi-drug resistant cases. The lead clinician is likely to need to spend 0.5–1 session per week on this, depending upon the numbers of local cases.

Assessment of patients for nebulisers and oxygen therapy   This is largely undertaken by a respiratory nurse specialist and the time spent by consultants on this work is encompassed in their normal outpatient commitments.

Specialist clinics   Many consultants offer dedicated clinics for patients with asthma, bronchiectasis and interstitial lung diseases. This may be in addition to their usual three clinics per week.

General practitioner x-ray reporting service   Some consultants provide a general practitioner X-ray reporting service. The commitment necessary for this is 0.5 session per week.

Examples of specialist services provided at a regional or supra-regional level

Cystic fibrosis   Patients with cystic fibrosis are usually cared for in large regional centres although some units provide the care for small numbers of patients and others share the care with the regional centre. Most large centres require the services of at least one whole-time equivalent consultant physician and supporting staff. Consultants supervising the care of only a few patients probably need to allocate one session per week for this work.

Lung transplantation   There are four centres in England where lung transplantation is undertaken. Each centre requires a consultant physician specialising in the assessment for and management of patients post transplantation. At least five sessions per week are necessary for this work.

Domiciliary assisted ventilation service – see above.

Occupational lung diseases – see above.

Services outwith the base hospital   Some consultants undertake outpatient clinics in hospitals other than their base hospital. This may be clinics in a city's central chest clinic or specialised clinics at another hospital. Some consultants provide general medical/respiratory clinics in outlying towns in rural areas. In general terms the time commitment for such clinics is included in their usual three clinics per week.

On-call for specialist advice and emergencies

Very few DGHs are able to provide continuous specialist advice from consultant physicians in respiratory medicine first on-call though specialist advice is usually available. Larger centres are able to provide such advice from on-call physicians and the frequency of the on-call work depends on the number of consultants in the unit or city if a city-wide service is provided.

The BMA has recommended the following allocation of sessions (measured as NHDs):

SpR available:	1 NHD each week
SHO available:	2 NHDs each week
Rota more often than 1:4	An additional 0.5 NHD each week

B Acute medicine

Most respiratory physicians have a commitment to the care of general medical patients admitted acutely. The on-call rota for such work varies enormously dependent on the number of physicians on the acute medical rota. In addition to being on call the consultant is required to undertake post-take ward rounds.

Approximately one-third of all medical patients who are admitted acutely have respiratory problems.

The BMA recommends the following allocation of sessions (measured as NHDs) to duties in acute medicine:

Rota Arrangements	
Rota less often than 1:5	1 NHD each week
Rota 1:4 or 1:5 with SpR	2 NHDs each week
Rota 1:3 with SHO	3 NHDs each week
Rota 1:3	4 NHDs each week

C Academic medicine

Each region should have an academic centre adequately staffed to co-ordinate regional teaching and research. This research should range from basic laboratory work through human studies to clinical trials. The BTS Research Committee and the BTS/MRC Clinical Trials Group currently run nation-wide multi-centre trails involving interested centres.

2   Work to maintain and improve the quality of care

This work encompasses duties in clinical governance, professional self-regulation, continuing professional development, education and training of others. For many consultants, at various times in their careers, it may include research, serving in management, and providing advice. All require consultant participation. Such work is described fully in Part 1 of this document. Its scope is summarised in the Appendix to Part 2. Management and advisory work are identified specifically in the Appendix.

WORKFORCE REQUIREMENTS

Currently (Oct. 2000), there are 542 consultants appointed in respiratory medicine in England and Wales. Because some work part time, this amounts to 488 WTEs, or 1 WTE per 108,490 people. The previous recommendation of the RCP workforce was 1:80,000 people, or 662 WTE consultants. The European average is 1 in 60,000. To achieve this would require 882 WTE consultants. Calculations show that delivery of a quality service in respiratory medicine would require 5 WTE consultants per 250,000 per head of population, the size of a typical DGH. To provide this, the specialty would need 1,060 WTEs, which, based on working practices in respiratory medicine in 2000 (RCP census), equates to 1,191 actual consultants.

The proportion of women in respiratory consultant posts is small at present, but set to rise dramatically. This is likely to have a significant impact on the ratio of actual consultants to WTEs, which currently is 1:0.79. By the time this target is reached, the total number of consultants required to reach this WTE target could be significantly greater.

The European Working Time directive of a 48 hour week, will have an enormous and legally binding impact on working practice. The RCP census 2000 shows respiratory consultants averaged 6 hours in excess of 48 per week. To meet the directive as well as to provide high quality service, the specialty would need to increase its consultant number from its present 542 to 1,508.

Calculation

General medicine on call   Most DGHs in the UK have twice daily rounds to cope with increasing numbers and to keep to College recommendation of >25 patients per post-take round. Therefore 12–14 NHDs per week are required for post-take ward rounds, depending on weekend arrangements. Most DGHs share this load between 5 specialties, working out at 3NHDs for post-take rounds. The specialty will typically be on-call 1:5 with SpR, equating to 2 further NHDs. Therefore, total NHDs for this activity = **5 per hospital.**

General medical follow-up clinics   A DGH of 250,000 admits 230–250 patients per week. The 1:5 share per specialty will therefore be 45–50 per week. The percentage requiring follow-up will vary across the country, typically 25–40%, ie 12–23 patients per week. Some need more than one follow-up visit, so the average DGH will need to provide 2 sessions of this activity per specialty (30 patients at 5 per hour). NHDs = **2 per hospital.**

Ward referrals   A DGH of this size typically generates 10 ward referrals per week in respiratory medicine from other specialties. At 30 minutes per new patient, the NHDs = **2 per hospital.**

Ward rounds   Each consultant needs to perform 2 rounds per week, in addition to the on-call rounds. These rounds take on average half an NHD, so total NHDs = **1 per consultant.**

Lung cancer   There are strict performance targets. The incidence of lung cancer varies across the population. In an average DGH of 250,000, 6 sessions of work are required. This includes MDT meetings, Lead clinician for lung cancer, and bronchoscopy sessions. Where the respiratory physicians provide chemotherapy, a further session is necessary. Therefore, NHDs = **6 or 7 per hospital for average DGH, depending on local arrangements for chemotherapy, but range will be 4–9 sessions.**

General clinics in respiratory medicine   A DGH of 250,000 will generate typically 750 non-cancer new referrals per year in respiratory medicine. A consultant is able to provide clinics for 40 weeks per year. The consultant sees 6 new patients per session, requiring 3.125 sessions per year. With a new:follow-up ratio of 4:1, allowing half the time for a follow-up patient, a further 6.25 sessions are required. NHDs = 9.5 Assuming that 2.5 **sessions of this activity is likely to be done by juniors or clinical assistants, allow 7 sessions for this.**

Specialised services within the specialty   These can be tabulated as follows:

Service	Sessions per DGH per week	Service	Sessions per DGH per week
Acute non-invasive ventilation	1–2	Home ventilation support	0.5
Terminal care	0.5–1	Hospital at home services for COPD	0/1, depending on availability
Nebuliser assessment	0–0.5	Occupational respiratory medicine	0.5
Oxygen assessment	0.5	Cystic fibrosis	0.5
Sleep	0.5 in addition to any clinics	TB treatment and contact tracing	0.5–2 depending on incidence
Pulmonary rehabiliation	0.5	**Total**	**5–10: assume 8 on average**

Not every hospital offers every service, but this provides a robust analysis, as hospitals performing less acute work offer a greater range of specialised services.

Conclusion   An average of 30 consultant sessions of work should be provided to service those sessions identified above as being on a per-hospital basis (ie all activity listed above apart from ward rounds). Each consultant will further provide 1 session per week in ward rounds. Assuming a 7 fixed-session contract, 1 of which is made up of the twice-weekly general ward rounds, then the 30 sessions of work requires 5 WTE consultants per DGH of 250,00 population.

Respiratory medicine: job plan of consultant

Direct Patient Care

Work in the specialty		Workload	allocated	NHDs
Inpatient	Ward rounds on base ward		20–25 patients	2
	HDU, ITU cover for acute respiratory failure		4–10 patients	0.5–2
	Referrals		1–15 patients	0.5–1
	MDT meetings		1–2 week	0.5
Outpatient	General respiratory	New pt Review pt	3 clinics/week. Per clinic General: New 2 pts/hour Review 5 pts/hour	3
	Special respiratory	New pt Review pt	Special: New 2 pts/hour Review 3–4 pts/hour Juniors see fewer depending on grade	
Specialised investigative and therapeutic procedure clinics	Bronchoscopy		6 patients per session	1
	Special bronchoscopy services		3 patients per session if offered	1
	Pleural disease: aspiration and biopsy		3–5 patients per week	0.5
	Pulmonary function testing		Supervision and reporting	0.5
Specialised services	Local: Lung cancer		Co-ordination and delivery of chemotherapy. 80/100,000 population	0.5–1
	Pulmonary rehabilitation		Variable locally	0.5–1
	Sleep related breathing disorders		Variable locally	0.5–1
	Pulmonary TB and contact tracing		Contact tracing, treatment variable locally	0.5–1
	Occupational lung disease		Diagnosis and specialist investigation	0.5–1
	Other			0.5–1
	Regional or supra-regional Cystic Fibrosis		Management and follow-up of patients. Variable between centres	10
	Lung transplantation		Planning, assessment, management and follow-up, variable between centres	5
Services outside base hospital	Included in outpatient service		As for outpatient service	Included in outpatient service
On-call for specialist advice and emergencies	Offered in limited centres		Variable	0.5

Work in Acute Medicine

On-take and mandatory post take rounds			Variable between hospitals. DGH 200,000 eg 20–35 patients per take. Two ward rounds per take. Clinic cancelled next day	Rota <1:5 = 1 Rota 1:4 to 1:5 = 2 Rota 1:3 = 3-4
Outpatient	General medicine	New pt Review pt	General: New 2 pts / hour Review 5 pts / hour	Included in the specialty clinics usually

Work in Academic Medicine

Clinical duties	As above		Variable depending on position	50% of each of above
Academic duties	Research Teaching Higher degree supervision Lectures Grant writing Study leave Administration			

Rheumatology

i   The specialty

Rheumatology incorporates the investigation, management and rehabilitation of patients with disorders of the musculoskeletal system, ie the locomotor apparatus, bone and soft connective tissues. Rheumatic disorders include inflammatory arthritis, autoimmune rheumatic disorders, soft tissue conditions (including injuries) osteoarthritis, spinal pain, chronic pain syndromes and metabolic bone disease. Rheumatology requires interdisciplinary knowledge and awareness of new research in internal medicine, immunology, orthopaedics, neurology and pain management, rehabilitation, psychiatry and professions allied to medicine. Training may also include specialist experience in paediatric and adolescent rheumatology, and sports medicine.

There is a common perception that all rheumatic conditions are chronic. This is not true. Mechanical and soft tissue lesions may be cured with relatively little input. Some conditions are acute (acute lupus, septic arthritis, rheumatoid vasculitis) may be life threatening and require emergency admission to hospital. Early and aggressive treatment of patients with rheumatoid arthritis may induce early remission and improve the prognosis. The introduction of new biologic therapies, requiring careful monitoring and documentation, has had a major impact on the work of rheumatologists.

ii   Organisation of the service

It is estimated that between 10–16% of all **primary care** (general practice) consultations are for rheumatic complaints. Some GPs with experience in rheumatology can provide an intermediate service for primary care colleagues, developing such a service in collaboration with local rheumatologists. Hospital (secondary care) services are provided in all districts, but their staffing varies (see below). Some consultant rheumatologists provide outreach services within primary care, but this is not usually an efficient means of provision and is generally not recommended.

Secondary care rheumatology services may be provided by consultants practising whole-time in the specialty, or by physicians who also have a general medicine component to their post and do acute medical takes. A few physicians do rheumatology and rehabilitation but this option for dual accreditation is no longer available to trainees.

Tertiary care services include specialist paediatric and adolescent rheumatology, and disease-specific clinics.

iii   Service considerations

Rheumatology is predominantly an outpatient specialty. Inflammatory joint disease occupies about 20% of new patient work, but over 80% of follow-up work. The majority of consultant rheumatologists have a large caseload of soft tissue injury, osteoarthritis, back and neck pain, chronic musculoskeletal pain (chronic pain syndrome, post-viral fatigue syndrome etc, and sports injuries). These are often dealt with on a 'one-stop' basis. Outpatient procedures undertaken by consultant rheumatologists include joint and soft tissue injections, and epidural injections. Some follow-up work and certain therapeutic procedures may be performed under consultant supervision by a suitably trained non-medical specialist practitioner, such as a nurse or physiotherapist. Inpatient care is often necessary for patients with serious exacerbations of disease, complications (such as infection) and for rehabilitation. Team working between rheumatology and orthopaedics is common, for example in the management of patients who have received joint replacements.

Beds should also be available for day patients, for administration of infusions, epidural injections, injections under general anaesthesia, biopsies.

It is essential that specialists monitor patients with inflammatory joint disease, especially rheumatoid arthritis (the most common). With the introduction of new drugs requiring regular detailed patient assessment, there must be adequate support for rheumatologists if they are to continue to provide the broad range of services outlined above. The development of specialist follow-up clinics run by metrologists and/or non-medical practitioners is thus inevitable.

Consultant rheumatologists must also have access to hospital beds. Beds for rheumatology patients should be in one ward, with junior medical staff, nursing and allied professional staff trained in the care of these patients. There is no absolute requirement for the ward to be medical. In some centres it may be more appropriate for rheumatology beds to be in dedicated specialty wards, or on orthopaedic wards. Bed provision should be determined according to local need.

iv Conjoined services

All rheumatology departments work closely with departments of:

- physiotherapy (to restore physical function, and educate in exercises and self-care);
- occupational therapy (for ongoing disability management, and specialist services such as hand function assessment);
- the wheelchair service;
- chiropody (which may be a combined service to cover a diabetic facility, as many problems are similar);
- dietetics (weight reduction may be an essential part of the management of osteoarthritis);
- surgical appliances and orthopaedic surgery (for joint replacement in particular).

There must be access to radiology facilities (including MRI) and ultrasound is used increasingly in diagnosis. In addition to general pathology there is a specific requirement for immunology services and for access to polarised light microscopy for examination of joint fluid samples.

Support for a rheumatology service

A rheumatology department must have adequate secretarial staff of sufficient experience and grade to be able to deal with patient enquiries and to arrange appointments. A rheumatology service has a large number of patients who are followed up over a long time, and may require urgent specialist access between appointments. Secretarial and medical records staff have important roles in co-ordinating this care. Likewise, whether the service has its own specialist nurse/therapy practitioners or not, it should have dedicated inpatient and outpatient nursing support. The development of departmental telephone help-lines is also considered important.

All of these improve quality of the service and patient satisfaction. Patients with chronic disabling disease are greatly reassured by the knowledge that they are looked after by a team that they know and can trust on a continuing basis.

The development of hospital intranets will enable the timely delivery of pathology and radiology results. Such information must be available to the clinician in the clinic. Electronic access to this, and the hospital Patient Information System, is essential. Where departments run their own database for monitoring follow-up patients, it should interface with the hospital system to avoid duplication of data entry.

Patient information

The patient is an essential member of the multidisciplinary approach to rheumatology and it is important that a rheumatology service has access to, or the ability to generate its own information. This may be in the form of leaflets or, on the basis that all clinicians have access to their hospital intranet, direcly generated from the department or hospital database. Internet access is also considered essential for access to specialty sites, Medline etc.

v   Outline of clinical work in the specialty

Rheumatology is predominantly an outpatient specialty. Outpatient clinics should be structured to ensure that patients have an adequate consultation time. Typically new patient appointments are divided into 'urgent', 'soon' and 'routine'. There may be special clinics, for injections for example, or for patients with early inflammatory joint disease, or for research. The waiting time for a new routine appointment should not exceed 13 weeks, and 8 weeks at the most for a patient with presumed rheumatoid arthritis.

Clinics are usually in a hospital. In some areas, outreach clinics in cottage hospitals or primary care settings may be appropriate. However, dispersed small-scale services may be inefficient, especially if complex or time-consuming monitoring is required and diagnostic and investigative facilities are not to hand. Most consultant rheumatologists perform domiciliary visits, although it is usually best for patients to see where there is immediate access to investigations. If they are too unwell to be seen in a clinic they are likely to be in need of immediate hospital admission.

vi   Quality standards

The concept of a quality driven service, with standards of care clearly defined in contracts, provides a framework in which the quality of rheumatology care for a community can be improved. Consultant rheumatologists should not work in isolation and should have appropriate support staff including specialist rheumatology nurses.

Standards need to be set in relation to:

▐   the referral system;

▐   outpatient clinics;

▐   rheumatology procedures;

▐   outpatient/daypatient treatment service; inpatient care;

▐   discharge from the rheumatology service;

- training of medical and nursing staff;
- availability of appropriate facilities and equipment;
- administration;
- information for, and education of patients; and
- storage and handling of medical records.

Timely access to a rheumatology service is essential. The National Institute for Clinical Excellence (NICE) has developed referral guidelines for back pain and osteoarthritis of the hip and knee. The guideline also recommends that any patient with suspected rheumatoid arthritis should have access to a specialist opinion within eight weeks. This is based on evidence that delayed initiation of disease-modifying drugs worsens the outcome.

vii Rheumatology and general (internal) medicine (G(I)M)

Some 20% of consultant rheumatologists have a commitment to G(I)M. The British Society for Rheumatology, in referring to the conflict between specialty care (largely outpatient) and general medicine (largely inpatient) argue, that no single-handed consultant rheumatologist should be expected to do G(I)M as well.

viii Academic rheumatology

Rheumatology has an active research base with many flourishing academic departments. Often these are closely associated with departments of immunology. There is concern that academic rheumatology may suffer if trainees with an academic intent have their training unduly prolonged by the inclusion of G(I)M. It is vital to maintain a flow of clinicians who wish to participate in academic activity. Recently a dearth of such applicants has led to the appointment of three non-clinical professors.

WORK OF CONSULTANTS IN RHEUMATOLOGY

1   Direct patient care

A Work in the specialty

The job plan below describes the work of a full-time consultant without a general medicine or rehabilitation interest. Workload figures are based on recommendations of best practice from the British Society for Rheumatology.[1]

A session is considered to be a notional half day (NHD). Job plans are based on a maximum part-time commitment of 10 NHDs per week. It is not expected that any consultant rheumatologist will have more than six fixed sessions per week.

Where the physician also has a general medical commitment and participates in the on-take rota, with post-take rounds, the number of clinics should be reduced accordingly. However, no consultant rheumatologist who provides a single-handed specialty service should be expected to have an acute general medical commitment.

Undergraduate and postgraduate teaching or supervision of specialist registrars will also reduce the number of patients seen by the consultant in a clinic.

Outpatient service

A full-time consultant rheumatologist would be expected to undertake 4–5 clinics weekly. This includes routine and special clinics and such activities as combined clinics with orthopaedic surgeons or paediatricians. The exact number will depend on other duties, the geography of the service (eg split sites), responsibility for a rehabilitation unit and administrative duties.

Ideally there should be 30 minutes for a new patient and 15 minutes for a follow-up appointment. If junior staff are shared with general medicine then they may be absent from clinics depending on their on-call rota; then clinic structure and numbers booked will need to take this into account.

Numbers of patients

New patients It is suggested that 6–8 new patients should be booked into a clinic for a single consultant. Five of these patients would be routine or soon bookings, with one always held for urgent cases. The optimum number depends on casemix.

Review clinics 12–15 review patients is considered a reasonable load for a single-handed consultant.

Mixed clinics One new patient takes the time of three review patients, depending a little on casemix.

The impact of additional staff in a rheumatology clinic Junior staff see fewer patients than a consultant, who must also oversee their work. It is recommended that for each GP Clinical Assistant, SHO or SpR, the number of additional patients booked per clinic should be as follows:

	New patients	*or* Review patients
GP Clinical Assistant	3 extra	*or* 7 extra
SHO/SpR	3 extra	*or* 7 extra
Experienced SpR	5 extra	*or* 12 extra

This allows time for supervision by the consultant.

When a rheumatology specialist practitioner (nursing or physiotherapy) is present, and can undertake monitoring or some procedures, a consultant can see more patients.

The impact of teaching in outpatient clinics

To allow for teaching in a clinic there should be about 25% fewer patients.

Inpatient service

Time should be allowed for day case work and for the small number of patients who admitted acutely ill with rheumatological conditions or the complications of such conditions or their treatment.

On-call work

Many large rheumatology departments have their own consultant on-call rota. This is essential if the trainees have on-call commitments. Even where consultant rheumatologists have no acute general medical responsibility, there are rheumatology emergencies. Some may be dealt with by the acute on-call team but consultant rheumatologist advice should always be available. Providing an emergency opinion service to A&E departments may also be an appropriate on-call activity.

B Acute medicine

See Section vi above.

C Academic medicine

See Section vii above.

2. Work to maintain and improve the quality of care

This work encompasses duties in clinical governance, professional self-regulation, continuing professional development, education and training of others. For many consultants, at various times in their careers, it may include research, serving in management, and providing advice. All require consultant participation. Such work is described fully in Part 1 of this document. Its scope is summarised in the Appendix to Part 2. Management and advisory work are identified specifically in the Appendix.

WORKFORCE REQUIREMENTS FOR RHEUMATOLOGY

On the basis that a full-time/maximum part-time consultant rheumatologist takes annual and study leave for a total of eight weeks in a year (and that it is not usual for locum cover to be provided) it has been estimated that each will be able to see about 616 new patients and 1,760 follow-up patients per year.[1,2] Bank holidays may cause further loss of clinic time. In addition, time for continuing professional development/medical education (CPD/CME) (100 hours per year) may also reduce availability to the service. For a hospital catchment population of 250,000 this requires the services of three whole-time equivalent consultant rheumatologists (33 NHDs), or about 1 per 85,000 population.

Based on data held by the Arthritis Research Campaign (ARC) Epidemiology Research Unit in Manchester there are currently 435 consultants with a commitment to rheumatology in England and Wales. This is equivalent to one per 120,523 of the population. Approximately 16% of rheumatologists also have a commitment to general medicine[2] and 16% have a commitment to rehabilitation. There are 55 academic posts. On the assumption that maximum part-time consultants work full-time, and allowing for sessional commitments to academic services, general medicine or rehabilitation (and allowing for part-time consultants), then there are 329 WTEs in rheumatology in England and Wales, equivalent to one per 159,335 of the population. To achieve one WTE per 85,000 population would require a total of 612 consultants. The current shortfall is therefore 283 (figures as at December 2000). This assumes that consultant rheumatologists continue to offer a broad service covering both inflammatory and non-inflammatory joint conditions. In this context it should be noted that the current curriculum for SpR training in rheumatology accommodates this wide range. It does not take into account any major changes of practice (for example, the monitoring of rheumatoid arthritis on a more detailed basis).

NOTES:

1. Figures for the numbers of consultant rheumatologists with a general medical commitment differ between the British Society for Rheumatology Manpower Register (which indicates 16% do rheumatology with an interest in general medicine) and the Royal College of Physicians' figures (which suggest 26%). This may be accounted for by differences between the in the questions asked. The College figure may be based on the number of consultant rheumatologists who take part in the general medical on-take rota without a formal commitment to General Internal Medicine otherwise.

2. *In 1999 there was insufficient information available to allow a more precise estimate of the workforce requirements in this specialty. This recent estimate provides a firmer basis for workforce planning but this too will need to be reviewed in the light of developments in practice and service delivery.*

WORK PROGRAMME

The following table gives an example of the work programmes of a consultant rheumatologist in a secondary centre (DGH). It includes the range of work undertaken, the recommended workload, and allocation of notional half days (NHDs).

Activity	Workload	NHDs
Direct patient care:		
Ward rounds and other inpatient work	4–6 inpatients; 2–6 internal referrals	1–2
Outpatients:		4–6
New patients	6 patients*	
Follow-up patients	12–15 patients*	
Specialist clinics:		
injection	6–12 patients	Fortnightly-quarterly
epidural	1–6 patients (requires additional support/monitoring)	depending on demand
ultrasound assessment	1–4 patients	
single disease clinics		
Work to maintain and improve the quality of health care:		2–4

*Figures modified by presence/absence of other staff (see main text)

References

1. *Musculoskeletal disorders: providing for the patient's needs. A basis for planning a rheumatology service.* British Society for Rheumatology 1994.

2. Symmons D, personal communication.

Appendix 1. Preparation of job plans

The specialty statements should inform and guide consultant physicians and their clinical and management colleagues in their discussions and negotiations. We recommend that each consultant should have a job plan which encompasses the information given below, ie it should seek to quantify both (a) direct patient care and (b) work to maintain and improve the quality of care, together with an account of the organisation, resources and facilities required. Each job plan should be predicated on a general job description and the duties and responsibilities of the post.

Content of a work programme:

1. Direct patient care
2. Work to maintain and improve the quality of care
   (a) Governance and self-regulation; education and training; research
   (b) Specific management and advisory work.

CONTENT OF A CONSULTANT'S WORK PROGRAMME

1. Direct patient care

Activity	Workload	NHDs allocated	Clinical support	Conjoined services
Work in the specialty[1]				
Inpatient work				
Outpatient clinics				
Specialised investigative and therapeutic procedure clinics				
Specialised services				
Work outwith the base hospital				
On-call for specialist advice and emergencies				
Work in another specialty[1]				
Inpatient work				
Outpatient clinics				
Specialised investigative and therapeutic procedure clinics				
Specialised services				
Work outwith the base hospital				
On-call for specialist advice and emergencies				
Work in general medicine[1]				
Elective inpatient work				
Outpatient clinics				
Work in acute medicine[2]				
On-take, and mandatory post-take rounds				
Outpatient clinics[1]				
Work in academic medicine				
NHS components [Identify as outlined above]				
University components [Identify as outlined below]				
Total NHDs allocated to these activities				

[1] Normally some of these sessions are fixed times each week.
[2] May be at fixed times, weekly or less often.

2. Work to maintain and improve the quality of care:
(A) Governance and self-regulation; education and training; research

Activity	Responsibilities	NHDs allocated	Resources required
Clinical governance[1]			Good data Effective IT Contracted or protected time
Lead clinician Clinical governance team member	Safeguard standards and improve the quality of care by supporting effective systems of clinical governance Advise on and contribute to the collection, processing and analysis of data necessary to support clinical and service audit		
Clinical audit (Might be incorporated into clinical teaching)	Participate in national or local programmes of audit of outcomes, process and structure Participate in critical incident review		
Professional self-regulation			Protected time Study leave
Protecting patients Setting standards of clinical practice	Safeguard professional standards of conduct and practice Safeguard the quality of the clinical consultation Contribute to the work of professional bodies in the development of clinical standards		
Continuing professional development	Maintain knowledge and skills in all areas of professional responsibility Participate in personal professional assessment Undertake annual review of job plans and performance appraisal		
Education and Training[2]			Protected (fixed) time Resources for teaching
Teaching undergraduates Structured specialist training Trust Tutor	Provide high quality tutorship and training Ensure ready access to information and evidence Ensure that continuing education, research and good practice are properly valued		
Research[3]			Protected time and resources for research
Undertaking research Oversight of clinical trials	Contribute to new knowledge on effective health care Safeguard the quality of research Safeguard the subjects of research		
Total NHDs allocated to these activities			

[1] May be at fixed times, weekly or less often.
[2] Formal teaching is normally at fixed times.
[3] Normally some of these sessions are fixed times each week.